REPORT DOCUMENTATION PAGE

Form Approved
OMB No. 0704-0188

Public reporting burden for this collection of information is estimated to average 1 hour per response, including the time for reviewing instructions, searching existing data sources, gathering and maintaining the data needed, and completing and reviewing the collection of information. Send comments regarding this burden estimate or any other aspect of this collection of information, including suggestions for reducing this burden, to Washington Headquarters Services, Directorate for Information Operations and Reports, 1215 Jefferson Davis Highway, Suite 1204, Arlington, VA 22202-4302, and to the Office of Management and Budget, Paperwork Reduction Project (0704-0188), Washington, DC 20503.

1. AGENCY USE ONLY (Leave blank)	2. REPORT DATE February 2005	3. REPORT TYPE AND DATES COVERED Final Report January 2002–December 2002

4. TITLE AND SUBTITLE
Drug and Alcohol Testing Results 2002 Annual Report

5. FUNDING NUMBERS
TM600/BB002

6. AUTHOR(S)
Randy Clarke,* Robert Gaumer,* Michael Redington, and Eve Rutyna

7. PERFORMING ORGANIZATION NAME(S) AND ADDRESS(ES)
U.S. Department of Transportation
Research and Special Programs Administration
John A. Volpe National Transportation Systems Center
55 Broadway
Cambridge, MA 02142-1093

8. PERFORMING ORGANIZATION REPORT NUMBER
DOT-VNTSC-FTA-05-05

9. SPONSORING/MONITORING AGENCY NAME(S) AND ADDRESS(ES)
U.S. Department of Transportation
Federal Transit Administration
Office of Safety and Security
Washington, DC 20590

10. SPONSORING/MONITORING AGENCY REPORT NUMBER
FTA-MA-26-5017-05-01

I0438931

11. SUPPLEMENTARY NOTES
* EG&G Technical Services, Inc.
  55 Broadway
  Cambridge, MA 02142-1093

12a. DISTRIBUTION/AVAILABILITY STATEMENT
This document is available to the public through the National Technical Information Service, Springfield, VA 22161

12b. DISTRIBUTION CODE

13. ABSTRACT (Maximum 200 words)

This is the seventh annual report of the results of the Federal Transit Administration's (FTA) Drug and Alcohol Testing Program. The report summarizes the new reporting requirements introduced for calendar year 2001, the requirements of the overall drug and alcohol testing program (the revised CFR Part 40 and CFR Part 655), the results from the data reported for 2002, and the random drug and alcohol violation rates (the percentage of persons selected for a random test who produced a positive specimen or refused to take the test) for calendar years 1996 through 2002.

The results of drug tests—for marijuana, cocaine, phencyclidine (PCP), opiates, and amphetamines—are compared with the results of alcohol tests for the various types of required tests. Statistics are presented for random, post-accident, reasonable suspicion, and pre-employment tests combined and for each individual test type. Those test results are further compared by employer type (transit agencies and contractors), employer size (large, small, and rural), employee category, FTA region, and the drug type.

Statistics on employees returned to duty and results of return to duty tests and follow-up tests are presented separately from results of the other four test types because return-to-duty tests and follow-up tests represent a different segment of the test population and not all employers offer rehabilitation.

14. SUBJECT TERMS
alcohol testing, drug testing, FTA-covered employees, random testing, safety-sensitive, violation rate, post-accident testing, return to duty

15. NUMBER OF PAGES
84

16. PRICE CODE

17. SECURITY CLASSIFICATION OF REPORT Unclassified	18. SECURITY CLASSIFICATION OF THIS PAGE Unclassified	19. SECURITY CLASSIFICATION OF THIS ABSTRACT Unclassified	20. LIMITATION OF ABSTRACT Unlimited

Preface

This annual report represents the cooperative efforts of many people. Extensive appreciation is extended to the U.S. Department of Transportation's Federal Transit Administration, the Volpe National Transportation Systems Center, and the following individuals who were instrumental in guiding this project and contributing to its success:

Michael Taborn
Director, Office of Transit Safety and Security
Federal Transit Administration

Jerry Powers
Drug and Alcohol Program Manager
Federal Transit Administration

Michael R. Redington
Program Manager/Transportation Industry Analyst
Volpe National Transportation Systems Center

METRIC/ENGLISH CONVERSION FACTORS

ENGLISH TO METRIC

LENGTH (APPROXIMATE)

1 inch (in) = 2.5 centimeters (cm)

1 foot (ft) = 30 centimeters (cm)

1 yard (yd) = 0.9 meter (m)

1 mile (mi) = 1.6 kilometers (km)

AREA (APPROXIMATE)

1 square inch (sq in, in^2) = 6.5 square centimeters (cm^2)

1 square foot (sq ft, ft^2) = 0.09 square meter (m^2)

1 square yard (sq yd, yd^2) = 0.8 square meter (m^2)

1 square mile (sq mi, mi^2) = 2.6 square kilometers (km^2)

1 acre = 0.4 hectare (he) = 4,000 square meters (m^2)

MASS - WEIGHT (APPROXIMATE)

1 ounce (oz) = 28 grams (gm)

1 pound (lb) = 0.45 kilogram (kg)

1 short ton = 2,000 pounds (lb) = 0.9 tonne (t)

VOLUME (APPROXIMATE)

1 teaspoon (tsp) = 5 milliliters (ml)

1 tablespoon (tbsp) = 15 milliliters (ml)

1 fluid ounce (fl oz) = 30 milliliters (ml)

1 cup (c) = 0.24 liter (l)

1 pint (pt) = 0.47 liter (l)

1 quart (qt) = 0.96 liter (l)

1 gallon (gal) = 3.8 liters (l)

1 cubic foot (cu ft, ft^3) = 0.03 cubic meter (m^3)

1 cubic yard (cu yd, yd^3) = 0.76 cubic meter (m^3)

TEMPERATURE (EXACT)

$[(x-32)(5/9)]$ °F = y °C

METRIC TO ENGLISH

LENGTH (APPROXIMATE)

1 millimeter (mm) = 0.04 inch (in)

1 centimeter (cm) = 0.4 inch (in)

1 meter (m) = 3.3 feet (ft)

1 meter (m) = 1.1 yards (yd)

1 kilometer (km) = 0.6 mile (mi)

AREA (APPROXIMATE)

1 square centimeter (cm^2) = 0.16 square inch (sq in, in^2)

1 square meter (m^2) = 1.2 square yards (sq yd, yd^2)

1 square kilometer (km^2) = 0.4 square mile (sq mi, mi^2)

10,000 square meters (m^2) = 1 hectare (ha) = 2.5 acres

MASS - WEIGHT (APPROXIMATE)

1 gram (gm) = 0.036 ounce (oz)

1 kilogram (kg) = 2.2 pounds (lb)

1 tonne (t) = 1,000 kilograms (kg)

= 1.1 short tons

VOLUME (APPROXIMATE)

1 milliliter (ml) = 0.03 fluid ounce (fl oz)

1 liter (l) = 2.1 pints (pt)

1 liter (l) = 1.06 quarts (qt)

1 liter (l) = 0.26 gallon (gal)

1 cubic meter (m^3) = 36 cubic feet (cu ft, ft^3)

1 cubic meter (m^3) = 1.3 cubic yards (cu yd, yd^3)

TEMPERATURE (EXACT)

$[(9/5) y + 32]$ °C = x °F

QUICK INCH - CENTIMETER LENGTH CONVERSION

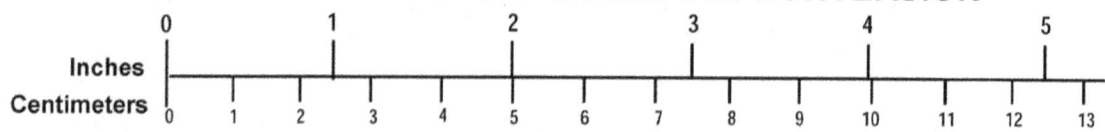

QUICK FAHRENHEIT - CELSIUS TEMPERATURE CONVERSION

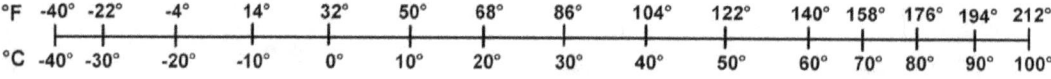

For more exact and or other conversion factors, see NIST Miscellaneous Publication 286, Units of Weights and Measures. Price $2.50 SD Catalog No. C13 10286

Updated 6/17/98

Executive Summary

Federal Transit Administration (FTA) regulations require that each recipient (both direct and indirect) of FTA funds (1) implement an anti-drug program to deter and detect the use of prohibited drugs, (2) establish a program to prevent the misuse of alcohol, and (3) report the results of its programs to FTA upon request. Compliance with FTA's drug and alcohol testing program is a condition of Federal assistance. Failure of a recipient to establish and implement a drug and alcohol testing program – either in its own operations or in those of an entity operating on its behalf – may result in the suspension of FTA funding to the recipient.

In 2001, FTA eliminated its requirement that all direct funding recipients report their drug and alcohol testing program data to FTA annually, and began using a stratified random sampling technique to select the funding recipients required to submit their data. This system was designed to produce an accurate representation of the overall transit industry, in lieu of universal reporting. The intent was to reduce the paperwork burden on a portion of the industry and to reduce FTA's tabulation and analysis effort. Sample sizes are determined for each of the three size groups[1] recognized by FTA (large, small, and rural) to ensure a distribution that accurately reflects the relative populations of the three groups. In 2002, 535 large employers, 36 small employers, and 237 rural employers were required to report their data.

2002 Testing Results

Results are summarized for the following areas:

- Violation rates (positive tests and test refusals combined) for random testing
- Accidents resulting in positive post-accident tests
- Positive test rates for four types of testing—random, post-accident, reasonable suspicion, and pre-employment
- Return to duty
- Random violation rate annual trends since 1996

Random Violation Rates

FTA considers random testing to be the most effective deterrent to drug use and alcohol misuse. The results of random tests also provide the best indication of the overall level of drug use and alcohol misuse, and are used by FTA in

---

[1] The population that surrounds the transit agency determines its size category. Large agencies are in areas of 200,000 or more, small is 50,000 to 200,000, and rural is less than 50,000. Transit agencies and contracted service providers are treated as individual entities in each group.

determining minimum annual random testing rates for the following year. For this reason, employers were requested to report the number of refusals to take a random test, as well as the number of positive test results. Accordingly, violation rates are presented for random tests. Violation rate is used here to refer to the number of positives and refusals combined per person selected to take a random test:

Drug violation rate[2] = (verified positives + refusals) ÷ (specimens collected + refusals)

Alcohol violation rate = (confirmed positives[3] + refusals) ÷ (screens collected + refusals)

Official Random Violation Rates for 2002

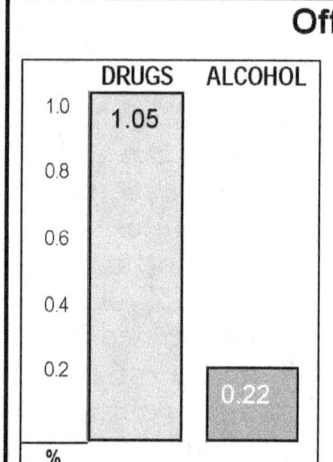

The graph at left shows the weighted "official" violation rates for random drug and random alcohol tests used by the FTA Administrator in determining the random testing rates for 2003.

Because the drug violation rate exceeded 1.0 and the alcohol violation rate was less than 0.50, both the random drug and alcohol testing rates remained at their current levels in 2003— 50 percent for drugs and 10 percent for alcohol.

The data that provide the statistical basis for the official violation rates are cited in the first paragraph on the next page.

The official violation rates used to determine the random testing rates for 2003 are not the actual percentages of the results reported. The results from the small and rural employers were given more weight than those from large employers because large employers have many more employees than small and rural employers. In 2002, 95.5 percent of the reported persons selected for a random drug test and 95.2 percent of those reported selected for a random alcohol test were reported by large employers. However, only 66 percent of the employers subject to the testing regulations were large employers. The same statistical procedure used to determine representative sample sizes was applied to the random test results.

The remainder of the data presented here reflect the actual reported (not weighted) test results.

The random violation rates for tests actually reported in 2002 were lower than the official rates for both drugs and alcohol. As shown in the graph at the top of the next page, the actual rates were 0.97 percent for drugs and 0.17 percent for alcohol. Results were reported for 82,584 persons who were selected for a drug

---

[2] For clarity in presenting the test results, the term "violation rate" is used differently here than in Part 655, where "violation rate" refers only to random alcohol tests.

[3] A positive alcohol test is a specimen with a confirmed breath alcohol level of at least 0.04.

---

test and for 26,478 persons who were selected for an alcohol test. Of those selected for a drug test, 732 had a verified positive result, and 718 refused to take the test. Of those selected for an alcohol test, 36 had a confirmed blood alcohol level of at least .04, and 13 refused to take the test.

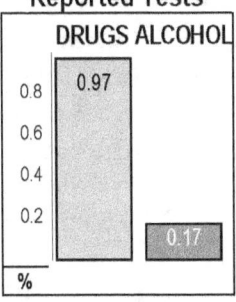

Actual Random Violation Rates for Reported Tests

As shown in the following three graphs, the random violation rates were much higher for contractors than for transit agency employees, and the drug rates were much higher for small employers than for the other two size categories while the alcohol rates were similar for all three size categories. More than 80 percent of those selected for a random test (both drugs and alcohol) were transit agency employees. More than 95 percent of those selected (both drug and alcohol) worked for a large employer.

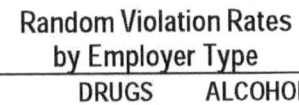

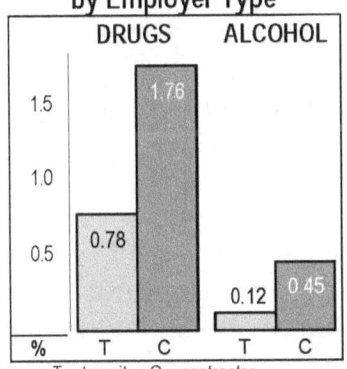

Random Violation Rates by Employer Type

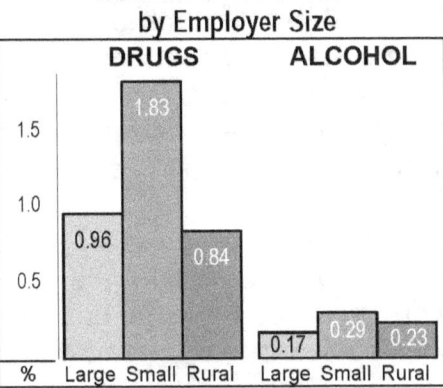

Random Violation Rates by Employer Size

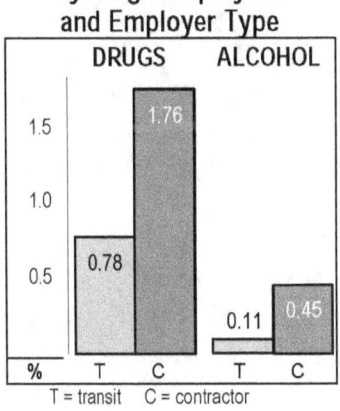

Random Violation Rates by Large Employers and Employer Type

As shown on the map at right, the random drug violation rate was lowest in the New England states (Region 1) at 0.62 percent, and was highest in the Middle Atlantic states (Region 3) at 1.32 percent. Only four regions had rates lower than the national average of 0.97 percent.

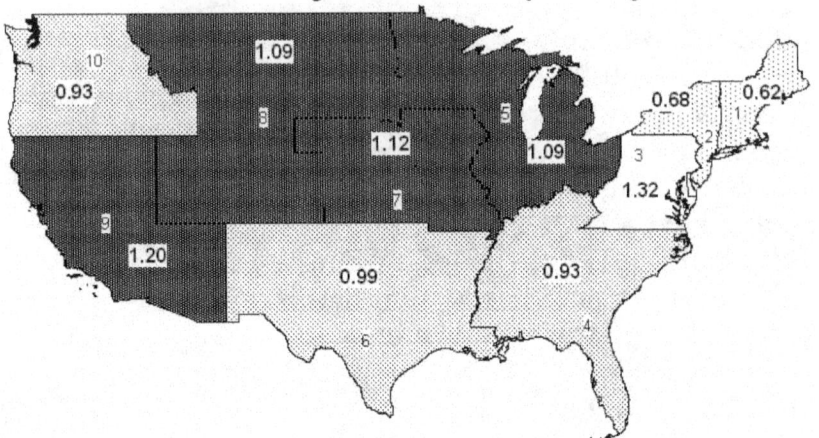

Random Drug Violation Rates by FTA Region

As shown on the map at right, the random alcohol violation rate was lowest in New York and New Jersey (Region 2) at 0.09 percent, and was highest in the central states (Region 7) at 0.37 percent.

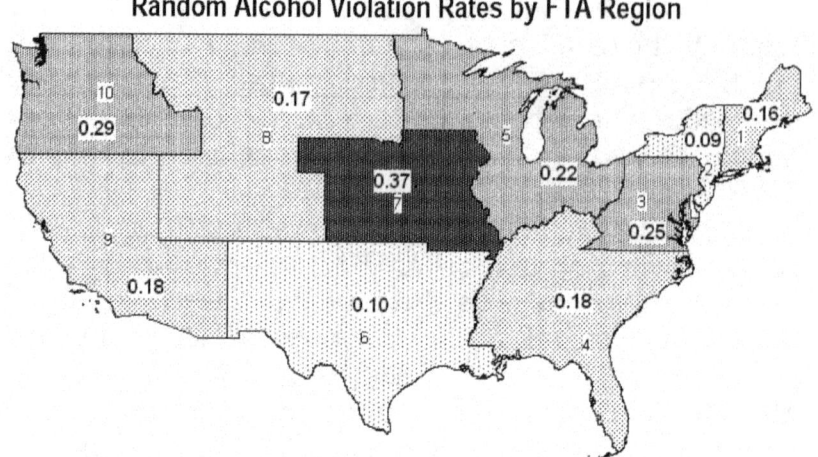

Random Alcohol Violation Rates by FTA Region

Refusal data were not collected by employee category or by drug type.

Accidents Resulting in Positive Post-Accident Tests

In 2002, employers reported 127 accidents that resulted in a positive post-accident drug test and 4 accidents that resulted in a positive post-accident alcohol test. These numbers when normalized to the entire number of employers required to test by FTA were 245 and 6, respectively. One of the accidents reported with a positive drug test resulted in one fatality.

Transit agencies reported 72 of the 126 non-fatal accidents with positive drug tests, and all 4 accidents with positive alcohol tests. All but 6 of the accidents with positive drug tests were reported by large employers. All the accidents with positive alcohol tests were reported by large employers. The positive drug test following the fatality was reported by a large transit agency in FTA Region 9.

Positive Test Rates[4] for Four Types of Testing

Because return to duty and follow-up tests represent a different segment of the test population (i.e., specimens produced by persons who have already been removed from duty for drug or alcohol violations and have completed a rehabilitation program) and not all employers offer rehabilitation, the data from those tests are not included in presentations of overall rates.

As shown in the graph at right, the reasonable suspicion positive rates were much higher than the random, post-accident,

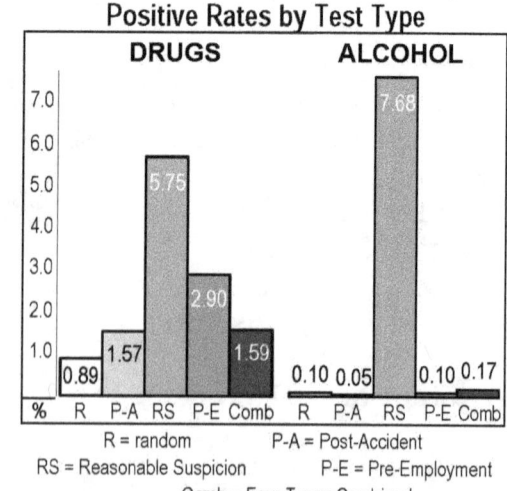

Positive Rates by Test Type

R = random   P-A = Post-Accident
RS = Reasonable Suspicion   P-E = Pre-Employment
Comb = Four Types Combined

---

[4] For clarity in presenting the test results, "positive rate" is used differently here than in Part 655, where it refers only to random drug tests and is the drug equivalent of the violation rate for alcohol.

or pre-employment rates for both drugs and alcohol. The random rate was lowest of the drug rates, significantly lower than the positive rates for any of the other three test types. The post-accident rate was the lowest of the alcohol rates.

As shown in the following three graphs, the positive drug rates for the four test types combined are more than two and one-half times as high for contractors as for transit agency employees, the alcohol rates are slightly higher for contractors, and small employers had the highest rates for drugs but reported no positives for alcohol. Of the 133,775 drug specimens collected for four test types combined, 95 percent were from large employers. Of the 45,601 alcohol screens collected, 95.5 percent were from large employers.

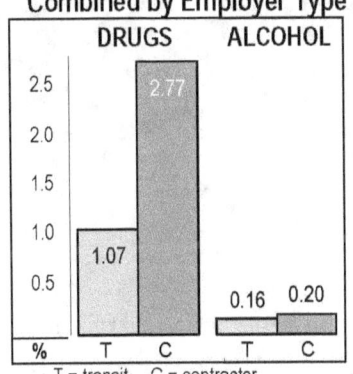

Positive Rates for Four Test Types Combined by Employer Type

T = transit   C = contractor

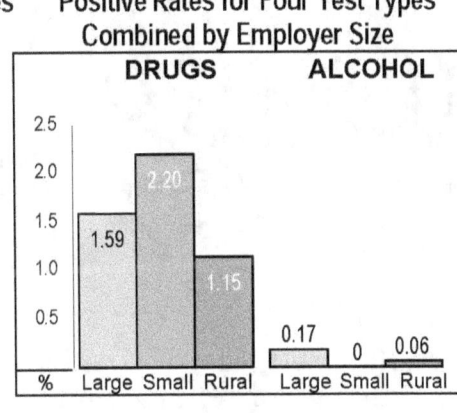

Positive Rates for Four Test Types Combined by Employer Size

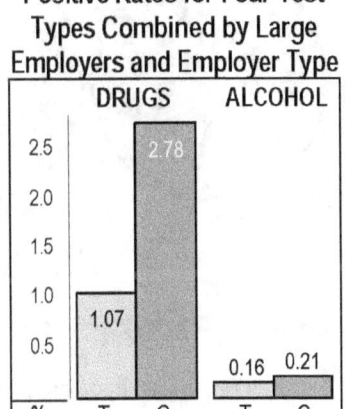

Positive Rates for Four Test Types Combined by Large Employers and Employer Type

T = transit   C = contractor

Because refusal data are not reported by employee category, random positive rates are presented below by employee category, as well as the rates for all four test types combined. The armed security personnel category had the lowest random drug rate and the lowest combined rate for drugs. The revenue vehicle operation category had the highest random rate and the highest combined rate for drugs. The revenue vehicle and equipment maintenance category had the highest random rate and the highest combined rate for alcohol.

Positive Rates for Random Testing and for Four Test Types Combined by Employee Category

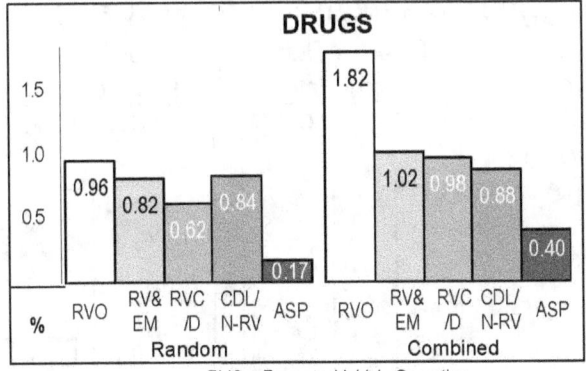

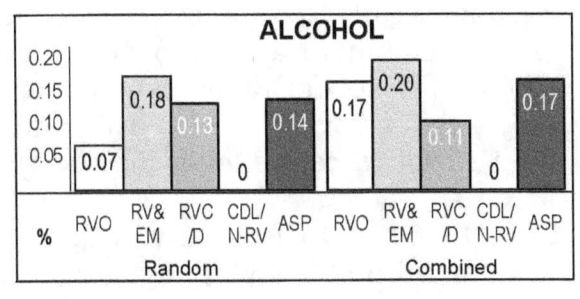

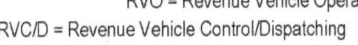

RVO = Revenue Vehicle Operation   RV&EM = Revenue Vehicle and Equipment Maintenance
RVC/D = Revenue Vehicle Control/Dispatching   CDL/N-RV = CDL/Non-Revenue Vehicle   ASP = Armed Security Personnel

As shown in the following charts, marijuana was detected as often as all of the other drugs combined in random testing, and more often than the others combined in reasonable suspicion tests and for all four test types combined. Marijuana was tested most often in post-accident tests, and cocaine was a close second. Cocaine was detected more often than the others combined in pre-employment tests while marijuana was detected in fewer than 20 percent of those tests.

Percentage by Drug Type of Total Drug Detections for Each Test Type

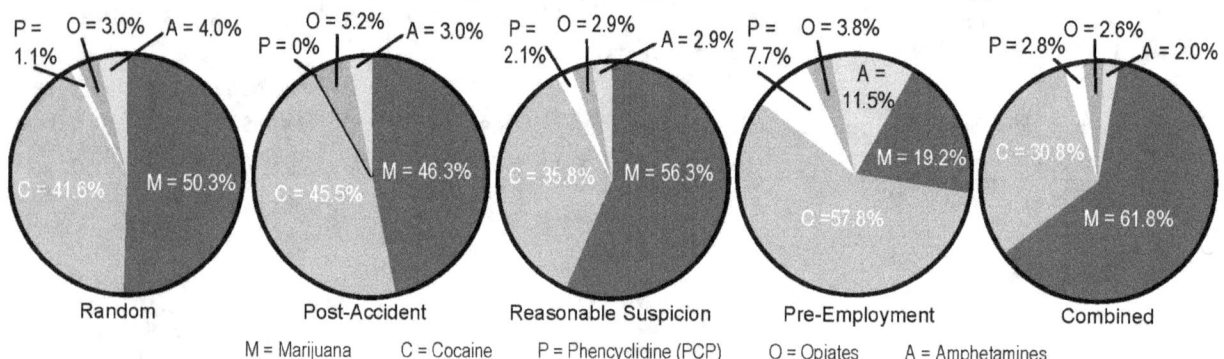

M = Marijuana   C = Cocaine   P = Phencyclidine (PCP)   O = Opiates   A = Amphetamines

Return to Duty Data

In 2002, employers reported that 358 safety-sensitive employees were returned to duty following a positive drug test or refusal, and 52 were returned following a positive alcohol test or refusal. These numbers when normalized to the entire number of employers required to test by FTA were 677 and 98, respectively.

Transit agencies returned 326 of the employees following a drug positive test or refusal, and returned 45 following an alcohol positive or refusal. Large employers returned 345 of the 358 returned following a drug positive or refusal, and returned 49 of the 52 returned following an alcohol positive or refusal.

Before being returned to duty, employees must complete a rehabilitation program and submit a negative test for the substance for which they were removed from safety-sensitive duty. Many employers require both a drug and alcohol return to duty test. The returned employees must then complete a series of follow-up tests (for the substance for which they were removed, or both drugs and alcohol) for a specified period following return to duty.

In 2002, 623 return to duty drug tests and 5,502 follow-up drug tests were reported. As shown at right, the return to duty positive rate was the higher of the two, and both were far less than 2 percent. Only 2

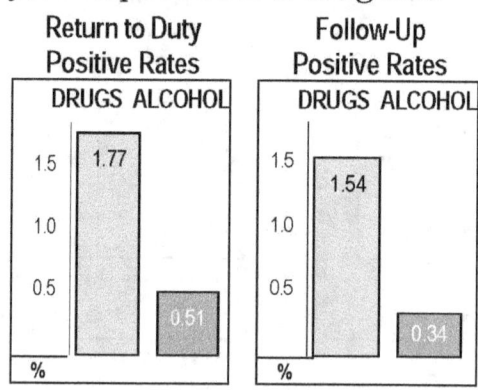

of the 396 return to duty alcohol tests reported were positive, and only 15 of 4,389 follow-up alcohol tests reported were positive.

The following six graphs subdivide the return to duty and the follow-up rates by employer type, employer size, and large employers and employer type combined. The follow-up drug test rates for contractors were slightly higher than those for transit employees for all employers and for large employers. The return to duty drug test rate for large employers was also higher for contractors, but the rate for all employers was higher for transit employees. There was only one return to duty drug positive reported by small employers and only one reported by rural employers. There was only one follow-up drug positive reported by small employers and only two reported by rural employers. Because these numbers are so low, the high rates for those employers are not statistically reliable. Thus, the drug test rates for small and for rural employers in both the return to duty and the follow-up graphs are presented on a separate scale from the other rates on those graphs. There were no return to duty or follow-up alcohol positives reported by either small or rural employers.

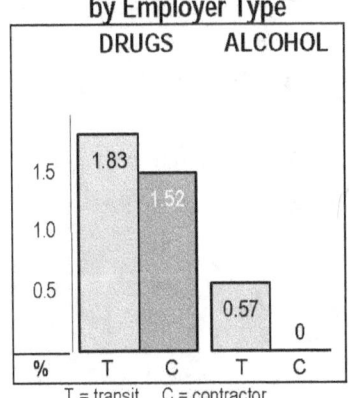

Return to Duty Positive Rates by Employer Type

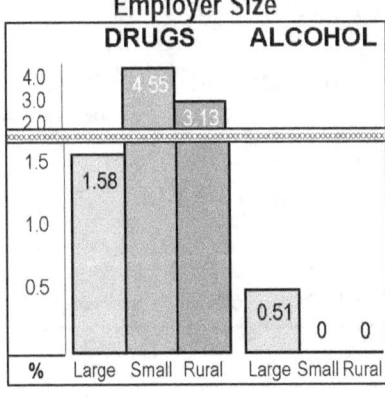

Return to Duty Positive Rates by Employer Size

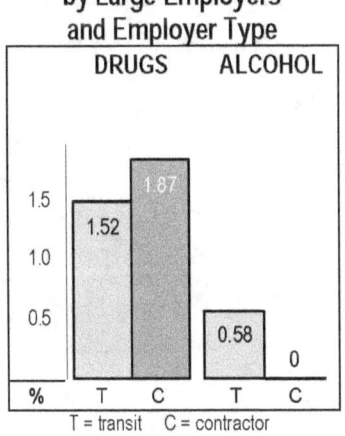

Follow-Up Positive Rates by Large Employers and Employer Type

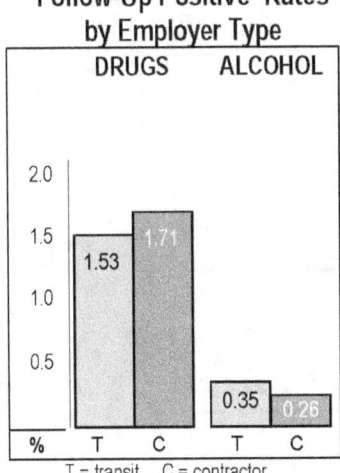

Follow-Up Positive Rates by Employer Type

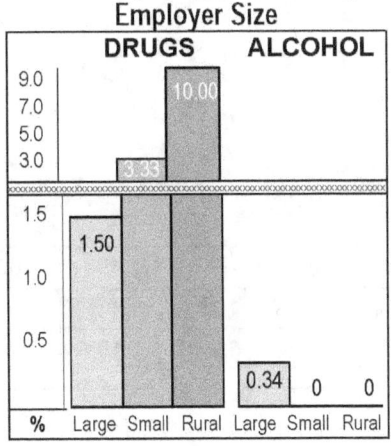

Follow-Up Positive Rates by Employer Size

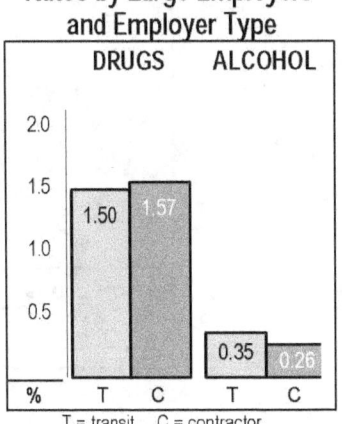

Return to Duty Positive Rates by Large Employers and Employer Type

Trends: 1996 Through 2002

Because the data reporting requirement changed in 2001, the only rates that can be reliably compared for each year of reporting (from 1996 to 2002) are random violation rates. As mentioned earlier, the results actually reported in 2001 and 2002 do not accurately reflect total FTA testing due to the large proportion of results reported by large employers. The results from random testing were weighted to obtain "official" random violation rates that reasonably estimate the rate for all persons tested, enabling reliable comparison with the years before 2001 when all employers were required to report. Weighted rates are not available for any test types other than random or any subsets of random testing.

As shown in the following graph, the drug violation rate rose in 2002, for the first time since employers in all size categories were required to report. The official weighted rate for 2002 rose above 1.0 percent, following its drop to 0.98 percent in 2001. Because it did not remain above 1.0 for the second consecutive year, the FTA Administrator did not have the option to reduce the random drug test quota for 2003. Although the official drug violation rate rose by more than 7 percent in 2002, equaling the rate in 2000 of 1.05, it was still nearly 35 percent lower than the rate in 1996.

As also shown in the next graph, the official random alcohol violation rate rose by more than 20 percent in 2002 (to 0.22 percent), equaling the highest rate (set in 1998). Despite its relatively high level, the 2002 alcohol violation rate remained well below the threshold of 0.50 percent for raising the testing rate from 10 to 25 percent.

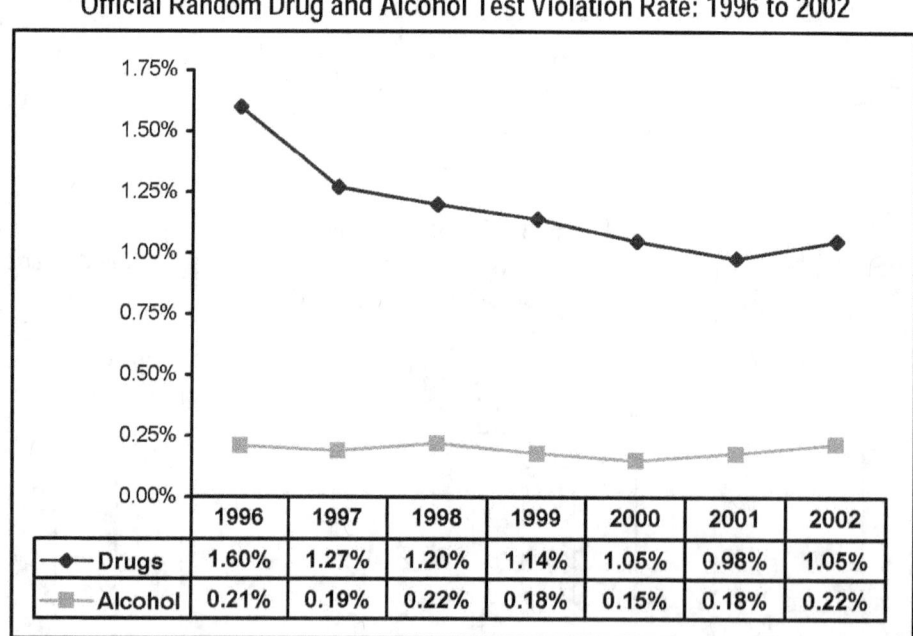

Official Random Drug and Alcohol Test Violation Rate: 1996 to 2002

	1996	1997	1998	1999	2000	2001	2002
Drugs	1.60%	1.27%	1.20%	1.14%	1.05%	0.98%	1.05%
Alcohol	0.21%	0.19%	0.22%	0.18%	0.15%	0.18%	0.22%

Table of Contents

1. Introduction

This report is the seventh annual summary of data submitted for entry in the Federal Transit Administration's (FTA) Drug and Alcohol Management Information System (DAMIS). The report summarizes data reported for calendar year 2002, and includes trend analyses based on the annual data submitted for calendar years 1996 through 2002. DAMIS contains the data from all the drug and alcohol tests conducted under FTA regulations between 1996 and 2000, but contains 2001 and 2002 data from only selected agencies, as explained in Section 1.2. DAMIS also contains the data from all the tests conducted by large agencies in 1995.

FTA regulations require recipients and subrecipients of funding under Title 49 of United States Code (U.S.C.) Sections 5307, 5309, and 5311, and 23 U.S.C. Section 103(e)(4) and their contractors to implement and maintain a program to deter and detect use of prohibited drugs and misuse of alcohol by safety-sensitive employees, unless the recipient is also an operating railroad regulated by the Federal Railroad Administration (FRA).

> *Section 5307 of 49 U.S.C.* refers to block grants to finance capital projects and the planning, improvement, and operating costs of equipment, facilities, and associated capital maintenance items for use in mass transportation.
>
> *Section 5309* refers to discretionary grants and loans for capital projects, new and existing fixed guideway systems, an efficient mass transportation system coordinated with other transportation systems, introduction of new technologies, enhancement of urban economic development or incorporation of private investment, and mass transportation projects to meet the needs of the elderly and persons with disabilities.
>
> *Section 5311* refers to financial assistance for non-urbanized areas.
>
> *Section 103(e)(4) of 23 U.S.C.* refers to grants to bus transit systems that operate on Federal-aid highway systems.

1.1 Regulatory Background

FTA issued its first drug and alcohol testing regulations on February 15, 1994 as two separate rules: 49 CFR Part 653, *Prevention of Prohibited Drug Use in Transit Operations*, and 49 CFR Part 654, *Prevention of Alcohol Misuse in Transit Operations*. The FTA rules were issued in response to *The Omnibus Transportation Employee Testing Act*, enacted by Congress in 1991. They expanded the minimum uniform DOT testing program requirements published earlier in 1994 in 49 CFR Part 40, *Procedures for Transportation Workplace Drug and Alcohol Testing Programs*.

The Omnibus Testing Act was intended to promote the health and safety of transportation employees and the traveling public. It required all DOT administrations to issue regulations requiring funding recipients to perform four types of testing of all safety-sensitive employees for five controlled substances and alcohol, and to establish a prescribed program of rehabilitation and follow-up testing for employees who are given the opportunity to return to safety-sensitive duty after testing positive or refusing to be tested. The Act also required recipients to follow the testing procedures established by the Department of Health and Human Services (DHHS).

DOT revised and reissued Part 40 in 2000. In 2001, FTA issued CFR Part 655, *Prevention of Alcohol Misuse and Prohibited Drug Use in Transit Operations*, to expand the revised department-wide minimum requirements to transit operations. Part 655 supersedes and combines Parts 653 and 654. The current Part 40 and 655 testing requirements are summarized in Chapter 2 of this report.

1.2 Reporting and Certification Requirements

Part 655.72 eliminated the requirement that all direct funding recipients report their drug and alcohol testing program data to FTA annually. It requires that recipients report their data only if requested by FTA. In 2001, FTA developed a stratified random sampling technique to produce an accurate representation of the overall transit industry, in lieu of universal reporting. The intent was to reduce the paperwork burden on a portion of the industry and to reduce FTA's tabulation and analysis effort.

In 2001 and 2002, sample sizes were determined for each of the three size groups recognized by FTA (large, small, and rural) to ensure a distribution that accurately reflects the relative populations of the three groups. The population that surrounds the transit organization determines the size of operation for each agency. Large, small, and rural organizations are categorized by a population of 200,000 or more, 50,000 to 200,000, and less than 50,000, respectively. In 2002, 535 large employers, 36 small employers, and 237 rural employers were asked to report.

Transit agencies and contracted service providers are treated as individual entities within each group. For example, an agency and two service providers it contracts with will represent three entities in the group's sample population. The samples were also selected using a random number generator or through a systematic process that ordered the entities by a specific criterion, such as alphabetic within state, to ensure that the sample was spread across all regions of the United States.

Recipients requested to report must do so on standard forms by March 15. All direct recipients must annually prepare and maintain a summary of the results of the programs that they oversaw during the previous calendar year. All direct recipients must also annually certify regulatory compliance of those programs, and submit the certifications to their FTA regional office. FTA operating funds are granted directly to most large transit agencies. All other operating grants are provided to the states or to metropolitan planning organizations (MPOs), which distribute the funds to individual transit agencies.

Some recipients and subrecipients (transit agencies funded by states or MPOs) rely on additional public or private entities to provide services in whole or in part. The states and MPOs must ensure the accuracy and timeliness of each report submitted by their subrecipients. All direct recipients must ensure the accuracy and timeliness of each report submitted by a service provider, operating or maintenance contractor, consortium or joint enterprise, or a third-party administrator acting on the behalf of a transit agency.

Failure of a recipient to establish a drug and alcohol testing program and to annually certify regulatory compliance and report information as requested, either in its own operations or in those of a subrecipient or an entity operating on its behalf, may result in the suspension of FTA funding to the recipient. Falsifying compliance information or certifications is a criminal offense.

1.3 Reporting Assistance

The required reporting forms are available in paper, on data diskette, and on the Internet. Copies of reporting guidance and reporting forms and diskettes are available from the DAMIS Project Office at (617) 494-6336. The FTA Safety and Security Clearinghouse can be reached at (617) 494-2108 for additional copies of this report, as well as previously published annual reports. Other technical assistance materials, including the *Implementation Guidelines for Drug and Alcohol Regulations in Mass Transit* and *Best Practices Manual: FTA Drug and Alcohol Testing Program,* can be obtained from the FTA Office of Safety and Security at (202) 366-2896 and on the Office of Safety and Security's Web site: http://transit-safety.volpe.dot.gov/damis.

1.4 Data Analysis and Validation

Data submitted for entry in DAMIS are subjected to extensive analysis and validation, both manual and automated. The process entails detailed review of the consistency and reasonableness of the data in each report, identification of errors or questionable entries, and resolution of any problems in consultation with the reporting agencies. This process enables detection and correction of errors of significant magnitude. However, some statistically minor errors may remain.

1.5 Organization of Report

The remainder of this report contains five chapters and three appendices:

- *Chapter 2* presents an overview of the current Part 40 and 655 testing requirements, including descriptions of safety-sensitive functions, the types of tests to be performed, and the substances to be tested for.

- *Chapter 3* compares the results of the required drug and alcohol tests listed in Chapter 2 and pre-employment alcohol tests. The results are further compared by employer type (transit agencies and contractors), employer size (large, small, and rural), the employee categories listed in Chapter 2, FTA region, and drug type.

- *Chapter 4* provides statistics on the number of employees returned to safety-sensitive duty in 2002 following a positive test or refusal, and summarizes the results of the tests (described in Chapter 2) that are required for such persons, using the same categories of comparison as in Chapter 3.

- *Chapter 5* presents random violation rates from 1996 through 2002, and compares selected rates for 2002 with those for 2001.

- *Appendix A* lists the terms, and their definitions, associated with the FTA drug and alcohol testing program.

- *Appendix B* lists the ten FTA regions and their headquarters.

- *Appendix C* presents by FTA region the number of accidents reported in which a transit agency employee or contractor tested positive in an FTA post-accident test.

2. Overview of Part 40 and Part 655 Testing Requirements

This chapter summarizes the requirements of the FTA Drug and Alcohol Testing Program (in Section 2.1) and describes in detail FTA safety-sensitive functions, the tests required by FTA, and the drugs that safety-sensitive employees must be tested for (in Sections 2.2, 2.3, and 2.4, respectively).

2.1 Overview of Required Testing Program

Employees who perform any of five safety-sensitive functions must be tested for five controlled substances in four circumstances. Such employees must also be tested for alcohol use in each of those circumstances except pre-employment, though employers may, and many do, require pre-employment tests per Part 40 testing procedures. An additional circumstance (return to duty/follow-up) is required for safety-sensitive employees who are given an opportunity to resume safety-sensitive duties after testing positive for drugs or alcohol or refusing to submit to a required test.

Safety-Sensitive Employee Categories	Test Types	Drug Types
Revenue Vehicle Operation	Random	Marijuana
Revenue Vehicle and Equipment Maintenance	Post-accident	Cocaine
Revenue Vehicle Control/Dispatching	Reasonable suspicion	Phencyclidine (PCP)
CDL/Non-Revenue Vehicle	Pre-employment	Opiates
Armed Security Personnel	*Return to duty/follow-up	Amphetamines
See Section 2.2 for a detailed description of FTA safety-sensitive duties.	See Section 2.3 for a detailed description of tests required by FTA.	See Section 2.4 for a detailed description of the drugs to test for.

*Required only for employees who test positive for drugs or alcohol or refuse to submit to a required test

Any employee who has a verified positive drug test, has a confirmed alcohol test result of 0.04 or greater, or refuses to submit to a test must be immediately removed from safety-sensitive duty. The employee must then be informed of the resources available for evaluating and resolving problems associated with prohibited drug use and alcohol misuse, including the names, addresses, and telephone numbers of substance abuse professionals (SAPs) and counseling and treatment programs. The employer then decides the disciplinary action to take. To return the employee to a safety-sensitive function, the employer must ensure that the employee successfully completes a course of treatment prescribed by a SAP and produces a negative return to duty test for drugs or alcohol or both, depending on the violation. Once returned to duty, the employee must continue a treatment program administered by the SAP, which includes a series of follow-up tests.

Additionally, an employee with a confirmed alcohol concentration of at least 0.02 but less than 0.04 must be removed from duty for at least 8 hours or until a re-test conducted by the employer shows an alcohol concentration of less than 0.02. If the employee is removed from duty for 8 hours, a re-test need not be administered unless the employee exhibits signs of alcohol use upon returning to duty.

Part 40 also prohibits use, manufacture, distribution, dispensing, and possession of all controlled substances by safety-sensitive employees. Furthermore, Parts 40 and 655 prohibit safety-sensitive employees from consuming alcohol in three circumstances:

- While performing a safety-sensitive function

- Four hours before performing a safety-sensitive function unless the employee produces a breath specimen with a concentration below 0.02 (Employees must be given the opportunity to acknowledge use of alcohol in the past 4 hours and to be tested when they arrive for duty.)

- Eight hours following an accident that meets FTA post-accident testing criteria (described in Section 2.3) or until an alcohol test is performed unless the employee's involvement can be completely discounted as a contributing factor to the accident and there were no fatalities

2.2 Safety-Sensitive Functions

The **revenue vehicle operation** safety-sensitive job category includes employees who operate a revenue service vehicle, regardless of whether it is in service and regardless of whether a fare is collected.

The ***revenue vehicle and equipment maintenance*** category includes employees who maintain revenue service vehicles or equipment. It also includes many maintenance contract employees who perform routine, ongoing repair or maintenance for FTA recipients and subrecipients that have employees, including supervisors, who perform or could be called upon to perform any of the FTA safety-sensitive functions. Maintenance contractors of 5311 funding recipients are not subject to the testing regulations.

Revenue vehicle control/dispatching includes employees who control the movement of revenue service vehicles. This function was much debated during the recent rule revision process because the title "dispatcher" covers a broad range of duties, not all of which are safety sensitive, throughout the industry. The key consideration is the type of work performed rather than a particular job title. FTA decided not to attempt a universal definition of "dispatchers" in Part 655. Instead, each employer determines whether its particular dispatcher performs or may perform a safety-sensitive function.

CDL/non-revenue vehicle includes employees not included in another safety-sensitive category who operate a non-revenue service vehicle (e.g., ancillary vehicle) that requires a Commercial Drivers License (CDL).

Armed security personnel are employees who provide security and carry a firearm.

2.3 Types of Tests

Random testing is considered by FTA to be the most effective deterrent to drug use and alcohol misuse, as well as the most reliable indicator of drug use and alcohol misuse within an agency and in the industry as a whole, provided it is unannounced and unpredictable. Thus, random testing is required to be conducted throughout all workdays and hours of service, and must be conducted at least once per calendar quarter. Selections for testing must be based on a scientifically valid random-number selection method, to ensure that all safety-sensitive employees have an equal chance of being selected for testing each time a selection is made.

In 2002, the number of random drug tests conducted had to equal at least 50 percent of the number of persons in the selection pool when selections were made, and the number of alcohol tests had to equal at least 10 percent of the pool. These percentages can be amended (per Part 655.45) by the FTA Administrator based on the combined percentage of positive tests plus test refusals, i.e.:

(verified positives + refusals) ÷ (specimens collected + refusals)

(confirmed positives + refusals) ÷ (screens collected + refusals)

The Administrator has the option to reduce a random drug or alcohol testing rate of 50 percent to 25 percent if the combined percentage of positives plus refusals is less than 1.0 for two consecutive calendar years. The Administrator has the option to raise a drug or alcohol testing rate from 25 percent to 50 percent if the combined percentage of positives plus refusals for the previous calendar year was at least 1.0. Additionally, the Administrator can reduce an alcohol testing rate of 25 percent or 50 percent to 10 percent if the combined percentage of positives plus refusals was less than 0.5 for two consecutive calendar years. Conversely, the Administrator can also raise a rate of 10 percent to 25 or to 50 percent if the combined percentage in the previous calendar year was at least 0.5 or 1.0, respectively.

It is important to note that the combined percentages used in 2001 and 2002 for determining the testing rate for the following year are not the actual percentages from all the tests reported. As mentioned in Chapter 1, only a portion of the employers were required to submit data in 2001 and 2002, and sample sizes were determined for each of the three size groups recognized by

FTA (large, small, and rural) to ensure a distribution that accurately reflects the relative populations of the three groups. However, because large employers have many more employees than small and rural employers, the distribution of the actual number of employees selected for random testing did not accurately reflect the relative populations of the three groups. More than 95 percent of the random test orders reported in both 2001 and 2002 were by large employers while only slightly more than 60 percent of the employers subject to the testing regulations are large employers. Consequently, the same statistical procedure used to determine representative sample sizes was applied to the random test results. The results from the small and rural employers were given more weight than those from large employers.

As shown in Chapter 3, the weighted "official" combined percentage of alcohol positives plus refusals was 0.22 in 2002 while the actual percentage was 0.19, and the weighted "official" combined percentage for drugs was 1.05 while the actual percentage was only 0.97. This distinction was particularly significant in 2002 because a drug rate below 1.00 percent would have permitted the Administrator to lower the drug testing rate to 25 percent. Based on the official rates, however, the random testing quotas for 2003 cannot change.

NOTE

Part 655 uses the term *"positive rate"* to refer to the concept of the combined percentage of random drug positives plus refusals, and defines the term as including only random drug test data.

Part 655 uses the term *"violation rate"* to refer to the concept of the combined percentage of random alcohol positives plus refusals, and defines the term as including only random alcohol test data.

For clarity in presenting test results, those terms are used as follows in this report:

"Violation rate" refers to the combined percentage of positive tests plus refusals for both drugs and alcohol.

"Positive rate" refers to the percentage of verified positive tests of the total number of drug specimens collected and to the percentage of confirmed positive tests of the total number of alcohol screens collected. Positive rate is used to refer to this percentage for all test types, including random.

In other words, in this report, *"violation rate"* includes refusals, and *"positive rate"* does not include refusals.

The testing rate for employers who belong to a consortium applies to the total number of safety-sensitive employees in the consortium's pool. As a result, some individual employers may not appear to meet the random testing requirement.

Post-accident testing refers to tests required following an accident involving a fatality or an accident that meets any of three other criteria and the employee's involvement cannot be completely discounted as a contributing factor: (1) when a person suffers a bodily injury and immediately receives medical attention away from the scene, (2) when any vehicle involved incurs damage requiring it to be transported away from the scene by a tow truck or other vehicle, or (3) the mass transit vehicle involved is a rail car, trolley car, trolley bus, or vessel and is removed from revenue service due to the accident.

Employees to be tested include the vehicle operator and any other safety-sensitive employee not in the vehicle whose performance could have contributed to the accident. Both drug and alcohol tests must be administered as soon as possible, but no later than 8 hours after the accident for alcohol and 32 hours for drugs. The results of a blood, urine, or breath test conducted by Federal, state, or local officials having independent authority for the test cannot be used to meet FTA requirements unless the employer is unable to perform a post-accident test within the required time period, the test conforms to the applicable Federal, state, or local testing requirements, and that the test results are obtained by the employer.

Reasonable suspicion testing refers to a drug and/or alcohol test that is ordered by a trained supervisor based on specific, contemporaneous, articulable observations concerning the appearance, behavior, speech, or body odor of a safety-sensitive employee.

Pre-employment testing refers to testing of candidates for a safety-sensitive position (including existing non-safety-sensitive employees as well as applicants for employment) and for employees who have not performed a safety-sensitive function for more than 90 consecutive calendar days, regardless of the reason, and were removed from the employer's random selection pool during that time. A negative pre-employment test for drugs is required by FTA as a condition for performing safety-sensitive duties under these circumstances. Pre-employment alcohol tests are not required but are permitted under Part 655 providing they are performed in accordance with the testing procedures in Part 40. The alcohol tests are included in the data presented in Chapter 3 because they are conducted per DOT standards and are required by many employers.

The Omnibus Testing Act required a negative pre-employment alcohol test, but FTA suspended the requirement on May 10, 1995, as the result of a U.S. Court of Appeals decision. FTA decided to allow but not require pre-employment alcohol testing in Part 655. All of the other eight DOT administrations with testing programs added this section to their rules.

Part 655 also eliminated the term "hire" in the pre-employment provision. Previously, employers were required to administer a drug test and receive a negative result before hiring an employee. FTA deleted the term to provide employers discretion to administer a pre-employment drug test anytime before an employee first performs a safety-sensitive function and before an employee returns to safety-sensitive duty after being removed from the random pool for an extended period. Part 655 also established a limit, 90 consecutive calendar days, on the amount of time an employee can be removed from the pool without a negative drug test before returning to work.

Return to duty testing refers to a drug and/or alcohol test that is required for a safety-sensitive employee who completes a course of treatment prescribed by a SAP after testing positive for drugs or alcohol or refusing to submit to a required test. A negative result for the type (drug or alcohol) of positive or refused test is required before the employee can be returned to duty. SAPs often require the employee to submit to both a drug and an alcohol test even if only one of the tests was at issue.

Follow-up testing refers to a drug and/or alcohol test that is required for an employee who is returned to safety-sensitive duty. The employee is subject to at least six unannounced tests for at least 12 months after returning to duty. The exact number and frequency of tests is prescribed by the SAP, who may order tests for up to 60 months after return to duty. SAPs often require the employee to submit to both a drug and an alcohol test even if only one of the tests was at issue. Follow-up testing is separate from, and in addition to, random testing.

Part 655 incorporates follow-up testing under return to duty testing (i.e., return to duty/follow-up testing) as one of five required FTA tests. It was previously listed separately as one of six required FTA tests.

2.4 Types of Drugs

Marijuana is derived from the hemp plant and comes in a variety of colors such as green, brown, and a gray mixture of leaves. THC or (delta-9-tetrahydrocannabinol) is the primary active chemical in marijuana. It is absorbed quickly into fatty tissues and stored for a long time. The potency and strength of the chemical causes people to use the drug for the mildly tranquilizing, mood and perception-altering effects it produces. The test for marijuana also includes its metabolites.

Cocaine is an addictive substance that comes from coca leaves, or is made synthetically. It appears as a white powder that is snorted, ingested, injected, freebased (smoked), or applied directly to the nasal membrane or gums. Cocaine acts as a stimulant to the central nervous system. It gives the user a feeling of exhilaration. The chemicals in cocaine trick the brain into feeling it has experienced pleasure, when in fact it has not.

Phencyclidine (PCP), originally developed as an anesthetic, has adverse side effects that limit its medical use to a tranquilizer for large animals. In people, PCP acts as both a depressant and a hallucinogen, and sometimes as a stimulant. PCP can cause distorted bodily perceptions and a feeling of disassociation where the mind feels separated from the body. These effects can be very upsetting to some people, who may panic as a result.

Opiates, also known as narcotic analgesics, include heroin, morphine, and codeine. They are derived from a sap taken from a seedpod of the plant, "papaver somniferum" (or poppy plant). General effects include sedation, slowed reflexes, raspy speech, sluggish movements, slowed breathing, cold skin, and vomiting. The synthetic form of opiates, known as "designer drug," is even more deadly and addictive.

Amphetamines include racemic, amphetamine, extroamphetamine, and methamphetamine. They are potent stimulants that may be swallowed, snorted, or injected. They induce exhilarating feelings of power, strength, energy, self-assertion, focus, and enhanced motivation. The need to sleep or eat is diminished. Amphetamines can induce a sense of aroused euphoria, which may last several hours. The body does not readily break down amphetamines. Thus, feelings are intensified and ephemeral. Subsequently, there is an intense feeling of mental depression and fatigue.

3. Drug and Alcohol Test Data

This chapter presents data from the four circumstances cited in Chapter 2 that must be performed by all employers subject to Part 655[1]: random, post-accident, reasonable suspicion, and pre-employment. Data from the fifth test type cited in Chapter 2 (return to duty/follow-up) are presented separately (in Chapter 4) from data for the other four test types because that test type represents a different segment of the test population—specimens produced by persons who have already been removed from duty for drug or alcohol violations and have completed a rehabilitation program—and not all employers offer rehabilitation.

As mentioned in Section 2.3, the results of random tests provide the best indication of the overall level of drug use and alcohol misuse, and they are used by FTA in determining minimum random testing rates for the following year. Thus, employers were requested to report the number of refusals to take a random test, as well as the number of positive test results, so the combined percentage of positive tests plus test refusals per person selected to take a random test can be determined. In this report, the combined percentage is referred to as the violation rate:

Drug violation rate[2] = (verified positives + refusals) ÷ (specimens collected + refusals)

Alcohol violation rate = (confirmed positives[3] + refusals) ÷ (screens collected + refusals)

NOTE

Given that only selected employers were required to report results in 2002, **the official violation rates used to determine the random testing rates for 2003 are not the actual percentages of the results reported**.

Employers requested to report in 2002 were chosen using a stratified random sampling technique based on the relative populations of the three size categories.[4] The results from the small and rural employers were given more weight than those from large employers because large employers have many more employees than small and rural employers. In 2002, 78,891 (95.5 percent) of the 82,584 reported persons selected for a random drug test and 23,672 (95.2 percent) of the 24,859 of those reported selected for a random alcohol test were reported by large employers.

---

[1] Part 655 does not require pre-employment alcohol testing. It is included in this chapter because many employers require it, and Part 655 requires that the data be reported if the tests are performed.

[2] For clarity in presenting the test results, the terms "violation rate" and "positive rate" are used differently in this report than in Part 655. See the text box in Section 2.3 for a full explanation.

[3] A positive alcohol test is a specimen with a confirmed breath alcohol level of at least 0.04.

[4] The population that surrounds the transit agency determines the size of operation for each agency. Large, small, and rural organizations are categorized by a population of 200,000 or more, 50,000 to 200,000, and less than 50,000, respectively.

However, only 66 percent of the employers subject to the testing regulations were large employers; 535 large employers, 36 small employers, and 237 rural employers were asked to report. The same statistical procedure used to determine representative sample sizes, mentioned in Chapter 1.2, was applied to the random test results.

Official Random Violation Rates for 2002

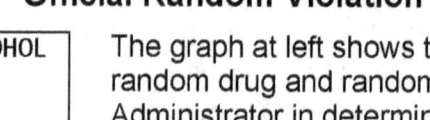

The graph at left shows the weighted "official" violation rates for random drug and random alcohol tests used by the FTA Administrator in determining the random testing rates for 2003.

Because the drug violation rate exceeded 1.0 and the alcohol violation rate was less than 0.50, both the random drug and alcohol testing rates remained at their current levels in 2003—50 percent for drugs and 10 percent for alcohol.

The data that provide the statistical basis for the official violation rates and the actual violation rates for the tests reported are presented in Section 3.1.

Employers were not asked to report refusal data for post-accident, reasonable suspicion, and pre-employment tests. The results of those tests are presented as verified positives for drugs and confirmed positives for alcohol. The verified/confirmed positive rates for random tests are included in the comparisons of positive rates by test type.

The results in the remainder of this chapter are expressed as rates (based on the actual data reported), where possible, or are normalized by each size category to represent the total number of employers. The actual number of instances reported is also presented to provide basis for the rate or normalization.

The data in the remainder of this chapter reflect the actual reported (not weighted) test results. Those data are presented in five sections:

3.1 Violation rates and supporting data for random drug and alcohol tests, subdivided by:
- Employer type (transit and contractor)
- Employer size (large, small, and rural)
- FTA region

3.2 Data on non-fatal accidents, fatal accidents, and total fatalities that resulted in positive post-accident drug or alcohol tests, subdivided by:
- Employer type
- Employer size

3.3 Verified/confirmed positive rates and supporting data for the four types of drug and alcohol tests, subdivided by:
- Employer type
- Employer size
- Employee category (safety-sensitive functions described in Section 2.2)
- FTA region (data only for totals for the four test types combined)

3.4 Verified positive rates and supporting data by type of drug for the four types of drug tests, including drug type rates and data by:
- Employer type
- Employer size
- Employee category

3.5 Non-positive alcohol violations:
- Alcohol specimens between 0.02 and 0.039 by test type, subdivided by employer type, employer size, employee category, and FTA region
- Non-test violations, subdivided by employer type and employer size

3.1 Random Test Violation[5] Data

The graph at right shows the actual violation rates for the tests reported. The accompanying table provides the statistical basis for the actual reported violation rates, and it includes the refusal rates. The actual data reported are subdivided by employer type and size and by FTA region later in this section. Refusal data were not reported by employee category.

Actual Random Violation Rates for Reported Tests

Persons Selected for Random Testing and Violations[5]

	Drugs	Alcohol
*Persons Selected	82,584	28,237
Refusals + Positives	803	49
Positives	732	28
Refusals	71	21
Refusal Rate	0. 086%	0.074%

*specimens collected + refusals for drugs
screens collected + refusals for alcohol

3.1.1 Random Test Violation Data by Employer Type and Size

The following three graphs present the reported random violation rates by employer type, by employer size, and by employer size and type, respectively. Each graph is accompanied by a table that provides the statistical basis for the violation rates. The tables also include the refusal rates.

---

[5] "Violation" refers to the combined number of refusals and positives. See footnote 1, on page 3-1.

Random Violation Rates by Employer Type

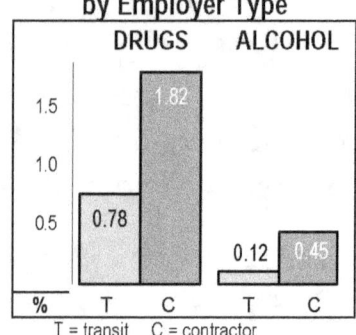

T = transit C = contractor

Persons Selected for Random Testing and Violations by Employer Type

	Drugs		Alcohol	
	Transit	Contractor	Transit	Contractor
*Persons Selected	67,073	15,511	23,369	4,868
Refusals + Positives	520	283	27	22
Positives	483	249	20	8
Refusals	37	34	7	14
Refusal Rate	0. 055%	0. 219%	0.030%	0.288%

*specimens collected + refusals for drugs
screens collected + refusals for alcohol

Random Violation Rates by Employer Size

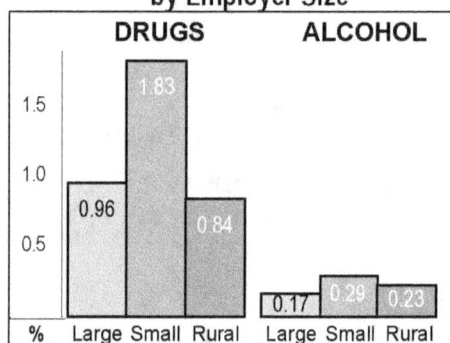

Persons Selected for Random Testing and Violations by Employer Size

	Drugs			Alcohol		
	Large	Small	Rural	Large	Small	Rural
*Persons Selected	78,891	1,200	2,493	27,034	339	864
Refusals+ Positives	760	22	21	46	1	2
Positives	700	17	15	27	0	1
Refusals	60	5	6	19	1	1
Refusal Rate	0.076%	0.419%	0.241%	0.070%	0.295%	0.116%

*specimens collected + refusals for drugs   or   screens collected + refusals for alcohol

Random Violation Rates by Employer Size and Employer Type

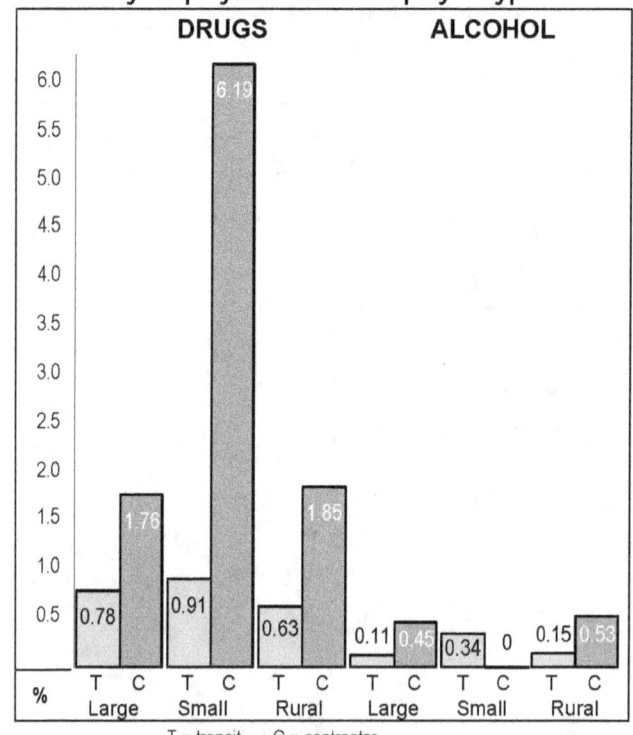

T = transit   C = contractor

Persons Selected for Random Testing and Violations by Employer Size and Employer Type

Drugs						
	Large		Small		Rural	
	Transit	Contractor	Transit	Contractor	Transit	Contractor
PS	64,023	14,868	990	210	2,060	433
R+P	498	262	9	13	13	8
P	464	236	7	10	12	3
R	34	26	2	3	1	5
R Rate	0.053%	0.175%	0.202%	1.429%	0.049%	1.155%

PS = persons selected (specimens collected + refusals)
P = positives   R = refusals   R rate = refusal rate

Alcohol						
	Large		Small		Rural	
	Transit	Contractor	Transit	Contractor	Transit	Contractor
PS	22,402	4,632	291	48	676	188
R+P	25	21	1	0	1	1
P	19	8	0	0	1	0
R	6	13	1	0	0	1
R Rate	0.027%	0.281%	0.345%	0%	0%	0.535%

PS = persons selected (screens collected + refusals)
P = positives   R = refusals   R rate = refusal rate

3.1.2 Random Violation Data by FTA Region

The following two maps show the random violation rates for drugs and for alcohol, respectively, for each of FTA's ten regions. The shading variations provide quick comparison. The exact rates are also included. The statistical basis for the violation rates is provided in the accompanying tables.

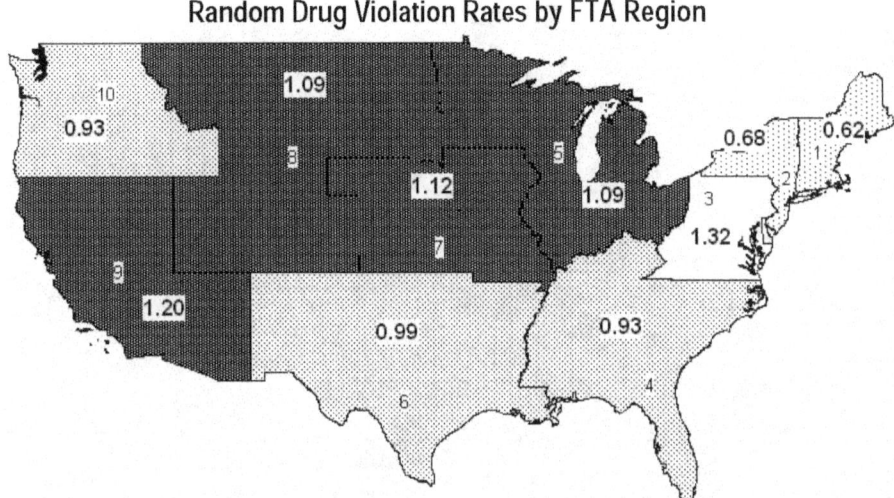

Random Drug Violation Rates by FTA Region

Persons Selected for Random Drug Testing and Violations by Region

Region	*Persons Selected	Verified Positives	Refusals
1	3,048	19	0
2	22,925	145	10
3	12,066	147	12
4	7,243	58	9
5	12,416	125	10
6	5,966	51	8
7	1,071	9	3
8	2,652	26	3
9	9,798	109	9
10	5,399	43	7

*specimens collected + refusals

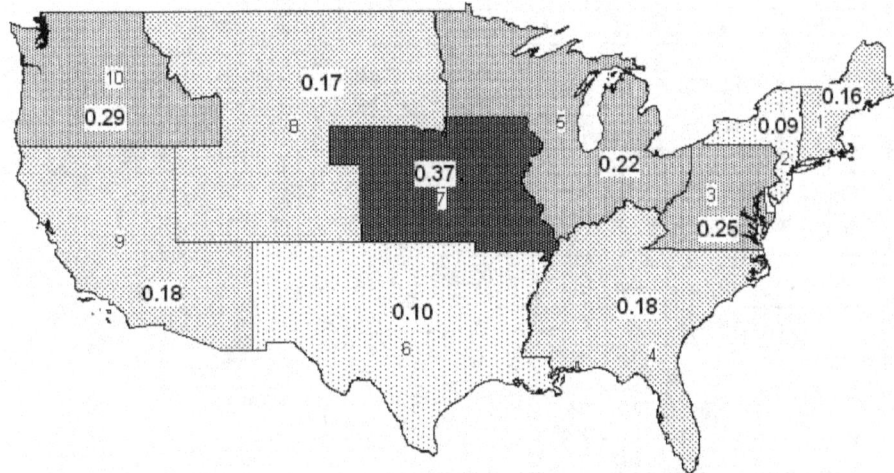

Random Alcohol Violation Rates by FTA Region

Persons Selected for Random Alcohol Testing and Violations by Region

Region	*Persons Selected	Confirmed Positives	Refusals
1	621	1	0
2	7,502	6	1
3	5,266	3	10
4	3,955	2	5
5	2,734	6	0
6	3,061	2	1
7	269	0	1
8	593	1	0
9	2,172	1	3
10	2,064	6	0

*screens collected + refusals

These data are subdivided by employer type and by employer size on the following pages. The drug violation rates by employer type, the drug violation rates for large employers, and the alcohol violation rates for large employers are displayed on maps. The statistical basis for the violation rates is provided in the accompanying tables. Because of the small sizes of their populations, the other rates appear in tables, along with the statistical basis for those rates.

Random Drug Violation Rates by FTA Region and Employer Type

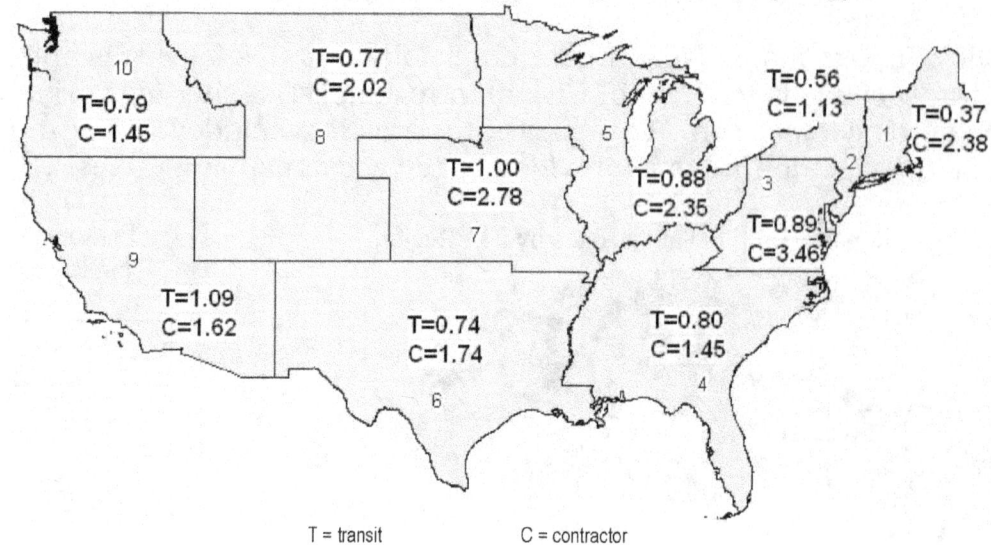

T = transit   C = contractor

Persons Selected for Random Drug Testing and Violations by FTA Region and Employer Type

Region	Transit			Contractor		
	Persons Selected	Verified Positives	Refusals	Persons Selected	Verified Positives	Refusals
1	2,670	10	0	378	9	0
2	18,429	97	7	4,496	48	3
3	10,071	88	2	1,995	59	10
4	5,865	42	5	1,378	16	4
5	10,625	87	6	1,791	38	4
6	4,468	28	5	1,498	23	3
7	999	8	2	72	1	1
8	1,959	13	2	693	13	1
9	7,694	79	5	2,104	30	4
10	4,293	31	3	1,106	12	4

Random Alcohol Violation Data by FTA Region and Employer Type

Region	Transit				Contractor			
	Persons Selected	Confirmed Positives	Refusals	Violation Rate	Persons Selected	Confirmed Positives	Refusals	Violation Rate
1	543	1	0	0.18%	78	0	0	0
2	6,004	3	1	0.07%	1,498	3	0	0.20%
3	4,465	2	1	0.07%	801	1	9	1.25%
4	3,365	1	3	0.12%	590	1	2	0.51%
5	2,158	6	0	0.28%	576	0	0	0
6	2,641	2	0	0.08%	420	0	1	0.24%
7	265	0	1	0.38%	4	0	0	0
8	406	0	0	0	187	1	0	0.53%
9	1,745	1	1	0.11%	427	0	2	0.47%
10	1,777	4	0	0.23%	287	2	0	0.70%

Random Drug Violation Rates by FTA Region and Employer Size—Large

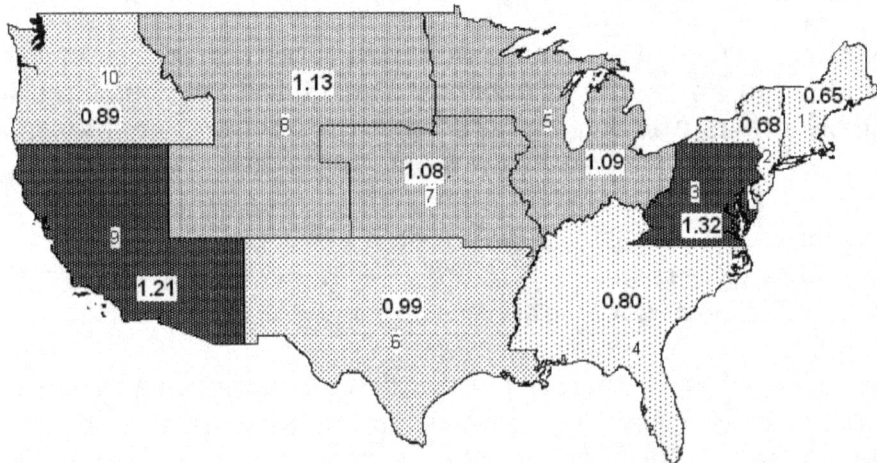

Persons Selected for Random Drug Testing and Violations by Region and Large Employer

Region	Persons Selected	Verified Positives	Refusals
1	2,939	19	0
2	22,925	145	10
3	12,066	147	12
4	5,738	42	4
5	11,280	116	7
6	5,881	50	8
7	1,019	9	2
8	2,556	26	3
9	9,682	108	9
10	4,805	38	5

Random Alcohol Violation Rates by FTA Region and Employer Size—Large

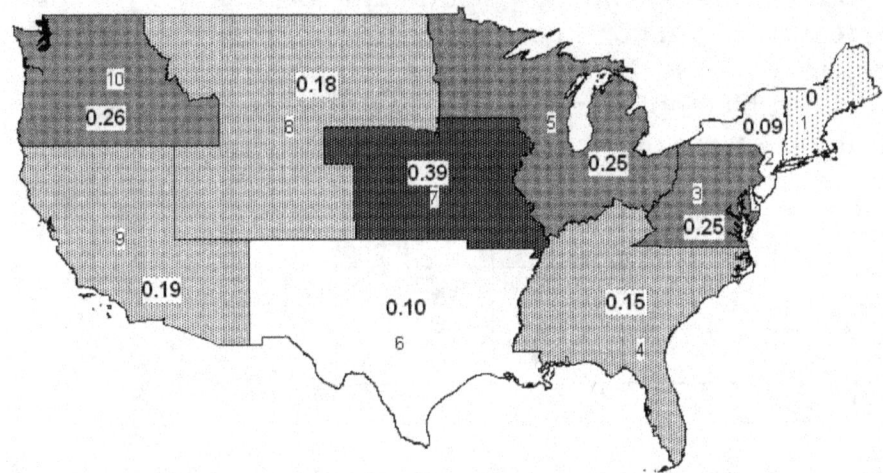

Persons Selected for Random Alcohol Testing and Violations by Region and Large Employer

Region	Persons Selected	Confirmed Positives	Refusals
1	606	1	0
2	7,502	6	1
3	5,266	3	10
4	3,347	2	3
5	2,425	6	0
6	3,020	2	1
7	259	0	1
8	565	1	0
9	2,147	1	3
10	1,897	5	0

Random Violation Data by FTA Region and Employer Size—Small and Rural

	Drugs								Alcohol							
	Small				Rural				Small				Rural			
Region	PS	VP	R	Rate	PS	VP	R	Rate	PS	CP	R	Rate	PS	CP	R	Rate
1	109	0	0	0	0	0	0	0	15	0	0	0	0	0	0	0
2	0	0	0	0	0	0	0	0	0	0	0	0	0	0	0	0
3	0	0	0	0	0	0	0	0	0	0	0	0	0	0	0	0
4	330	9	2	3.33%	1,175	7	3	0.85%	127	0	1	0.79%	481	0	1	0
5	412	6	2	1.94%	724	3	1	0.55%	93	0	0	0	216	0	0	0
6	85	1	0	1.18%	0	0	0	0	41	0	0	0	0	0	0	0
7	52	0	1	1.92%	0	0	0	0	10	0	0	0	0	0	0	0
8	96	0	0	0	0	0	0	0	28	0	0	0	0	0	0	0
9	116	1	0	0.86%	0	0	0	0	25	0	0	0	0	0	0	0
10	0	0	0	0	594	5	2	1.18%	0	0	0	0	167	1	0	0.60%

PS = persons selected   VP = verified positives   R = refusals   Rate = violation rate   CP = confirmed positives

3.2 Accident and Fatality Data Associated with Positive Post-Accident Tests

Data are presented for the number of accidents in which a transit agency employee or contractor tested positive in an FTA post-accident test. Data are presented for both drug tests and alcohol tests, though it should be noted that one person may test positive for both drugs and alcohol and that most employers test the employee for both drugs and alcohol. Thus, the numbers for drugs and alcohol cannot be added to obtain the total number of persons who tested positive. Data were not reported on the total number of persons testing positive in a post-accident test or for persons testing positive for both drugs and alcohol.

Because these accident and fatality numbers cannot be expressed as a rate, the number of instances reported have been normalized for the total number of employers by each size category. The first table below presents these statistics for the number of non-fatal accidents, fatal accidents, and total fatalities when a positive drug test resulted and when a positive alcohol test resulted. The next two tables subdivide those data by employer type and employer size, respectively. The data reported cannot be normalized by FTA region. The actual number of instances reported by region are presented in Appendix C; those numbers are also subdivided by employer type and by employer size. These accident and fatality numbers were not reported by employee category.

Accidents and Fatalities Resulting in Post-Accident Positives

	Drugs		Alcohol	
	Normalized	Reported	Normalized	Reported
Non-Fatal Accidents	244	126	6	4
Fatal Accidents	1	1	0	0
Total Fatalities	1	1	0	0

Accidents and Fatalities Resulting in Post-Accident Positives by Employer Type

	Drugs				Alcohol			
	Normalized		Reported		Normalized		Reported	
	Transit	Contractor	Transit	Contractor	Transit	Contractor	Transit	Contractor
Non-Fatal Accidents	139	105	72	54	6	0	4	0
Fatal Accidents	1	0	1	0	0	0	0	0
Total Fatalities	1	0	1	0	0	0	0	0

Accidents and Fatalities Resulting in Post-Accident Positives by Employer Size

	Drugs						Alcohol					
	Normalized			Reported			Normalized			Reported		
	Large	Small	Rural	Large	Small	Rural	Large	Small	Rural	Large	Small	Rural
Non-Fatal Accidents	195	31	18	120	3	3	6	0	0	4	0	0
Fatal Accidents	1	0	0	1	0	0	0	0	0	0	0	0
Total Fatalities	1	0	0	1	0	0	0	0	0	0	0	0

3.3 Data for Four Test Types

The two charts that follow compare the percentages of total verified drug positives and percentages of total drug specimens reported in 2002 for each of the four test types: random, post-accident, reasonable suspicion, and pre-employment. Those charts are followed by two charts that compare the percentages of total confirmed alcohol positives and percentages of total alcohol screens reported in 2002.

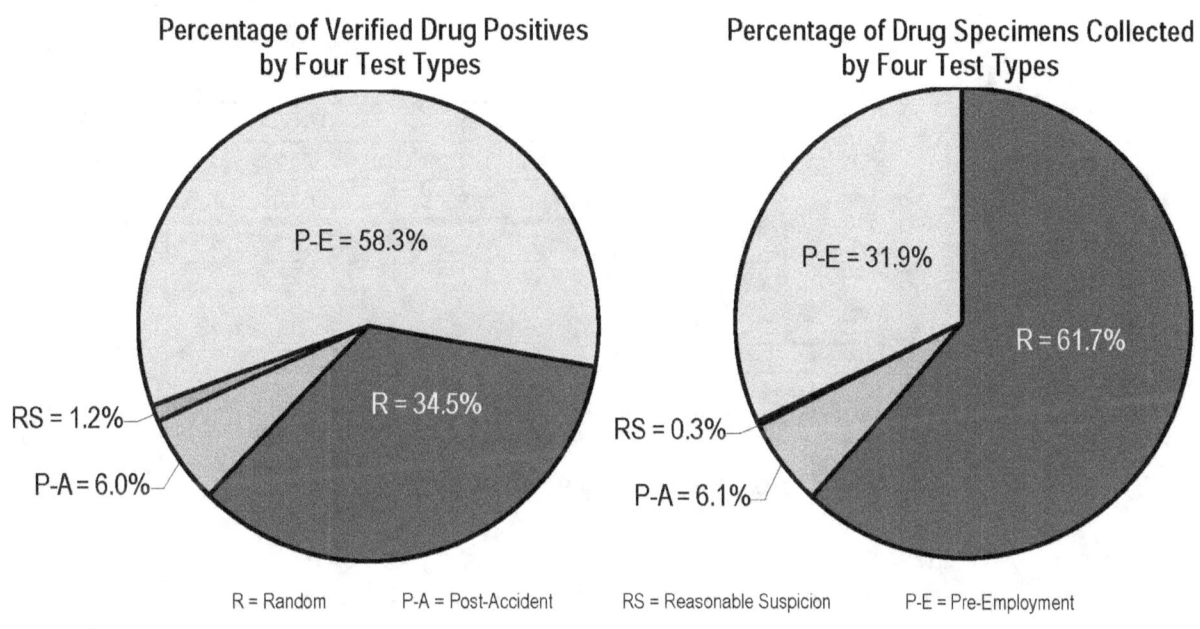

Percentage of Verified Drug Positives by Four Test Types

P-E = 58.3%
R = 34.5%
RS = 1.2%
P-A = 6.0%

Percentage of Drug Specimens Collected by Four Test Types

P-E = 31.9%
R = 61.7%
RS = 0.3%
P-A = 6.1%

R = Random   P-A = Post-Accident   RS = Reasonable Suspicion   P-E = Pre-Employment

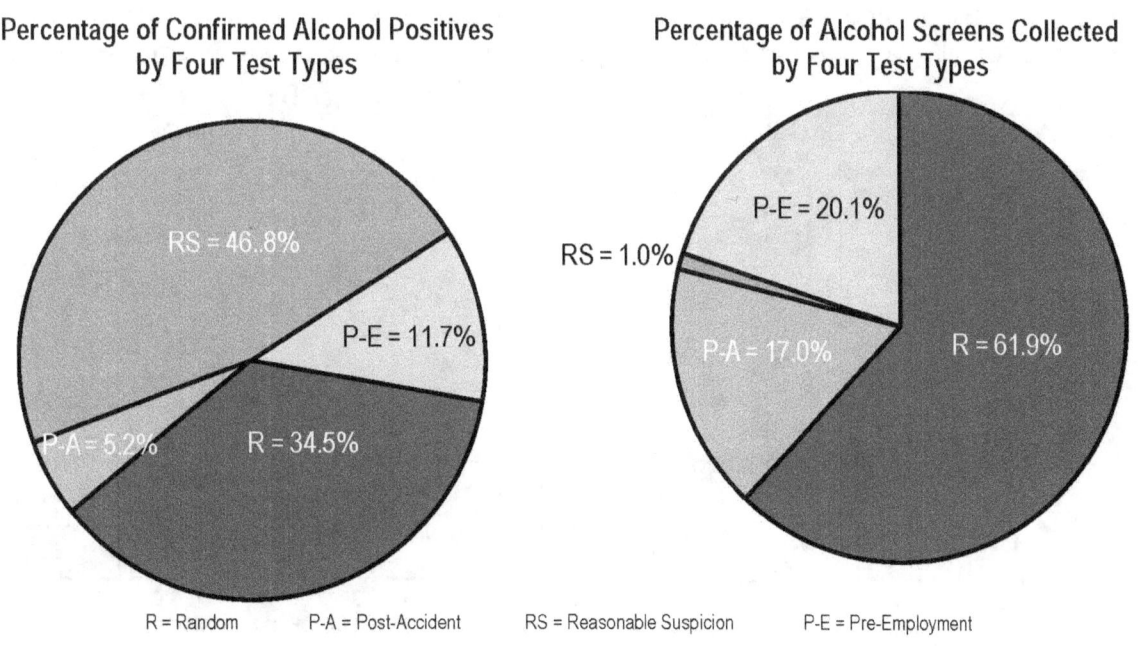

Percentage of Confirmed Alcohol Positives by Four Test Types

RS = 46..8%
P-E = 11.7%
P-A = 5.2%
R = 34.5%

Percentage of Alcohol Screens Collected by Four Test Types

P-E = 20.1%
RS = 1.0%
P-A = 17.0%
R = 61.9%

R = Random   P-A = Post-Accident   RS = Reasonable Suspicion   P-E = Pre-Employment

The positive rates for each of the four types and for the four types combined, for both drug tests and alcohol tests, are presented in the following graph. The accompanying table provides the statistical basis for the positive rates. These data are subdivided by employer type and size, by employee category, and by FTA region later in this section.

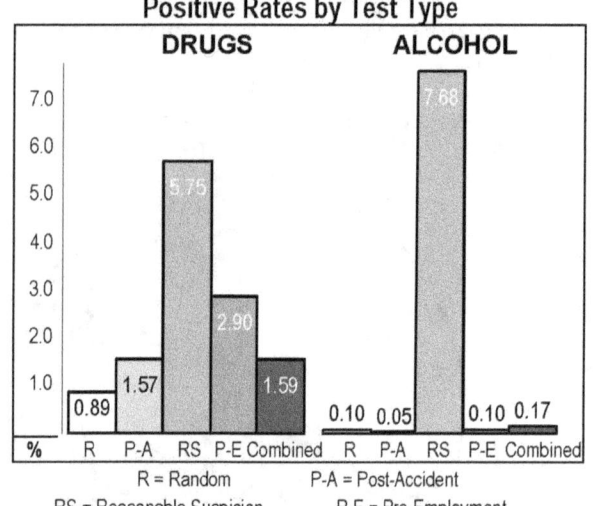

Positive Rates by Test Type

R = Random   P-A = Post-Accident
RS = Reasonable Suspicion   P-E = Pre-Employment

Specimens/Screens Collected and Positives by Test Type

	Drugs		Alcohol	
	Specimens Collected	Verified Positives	Screens	Confirmed Positives
Random	82,513	732	28,216	28
Post-Accident	8,160	128	7,759	4
Reasonable Suspicion	452	26	469	36
Pre-Employment	42,650	1,236	9,157	9
Total	133,775	2,122	45,601	77

3.3.1 Data for Four Test Types by Employer Type and Size

The data above are subdivided by employer type, by employer size, and by employer size and type, respectively, in this section. The rates for each data set are shown in a separate pair of graphs. Each graph pair is followed by a table that provides the statistical basis for the rates. Because all of the alcohol rates except reasonable suspicion are 0.2 percent or less, the space below "0.2" in each alcohol graph is expanded under the divider line to allow greater clarity.

Positive Rates by Test Type and Employer Type

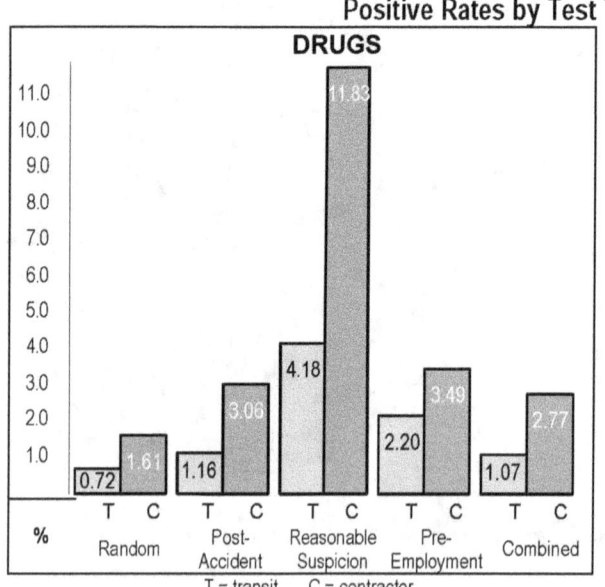

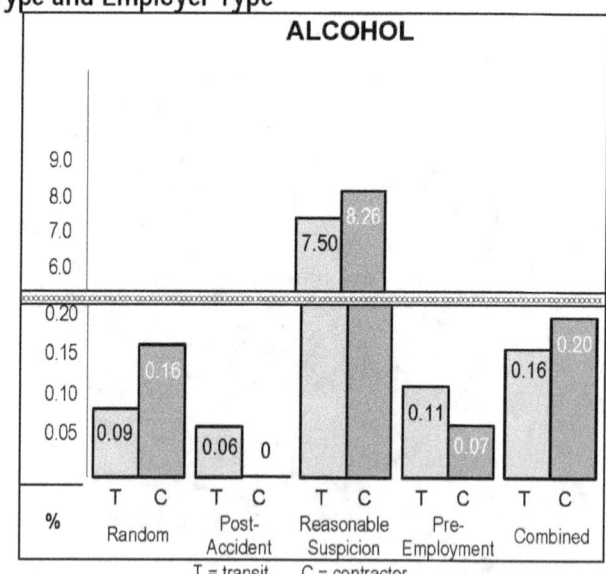

T = transit   C = contractor

Specimens/Screens Collected and Positives by Test Type and Employer Type

	Drugs				Alcohol			
	Transit		Contractor		Transit		Contractor	
	Specimens Collected	Verified Positives	Specimens Collected	Verified Positives	Screens	Confirmed Positives	Screens	Confirmed Positives
Random	67,036	483	15,477	249	23,362	20	4,854	8
Post-Accident	6,397	74	1,763	54	6222	4	1,537	0
Reasonable Suspicion	359	15	93	11	360	27	109	9
Pre-Employment	19,471	428	23,179	808	6,149	7	3,008	2
Total	93,263	1,000	40,512	1,122	36,093	58	9,508	19

Positive Rates by Test Type and Employer Size

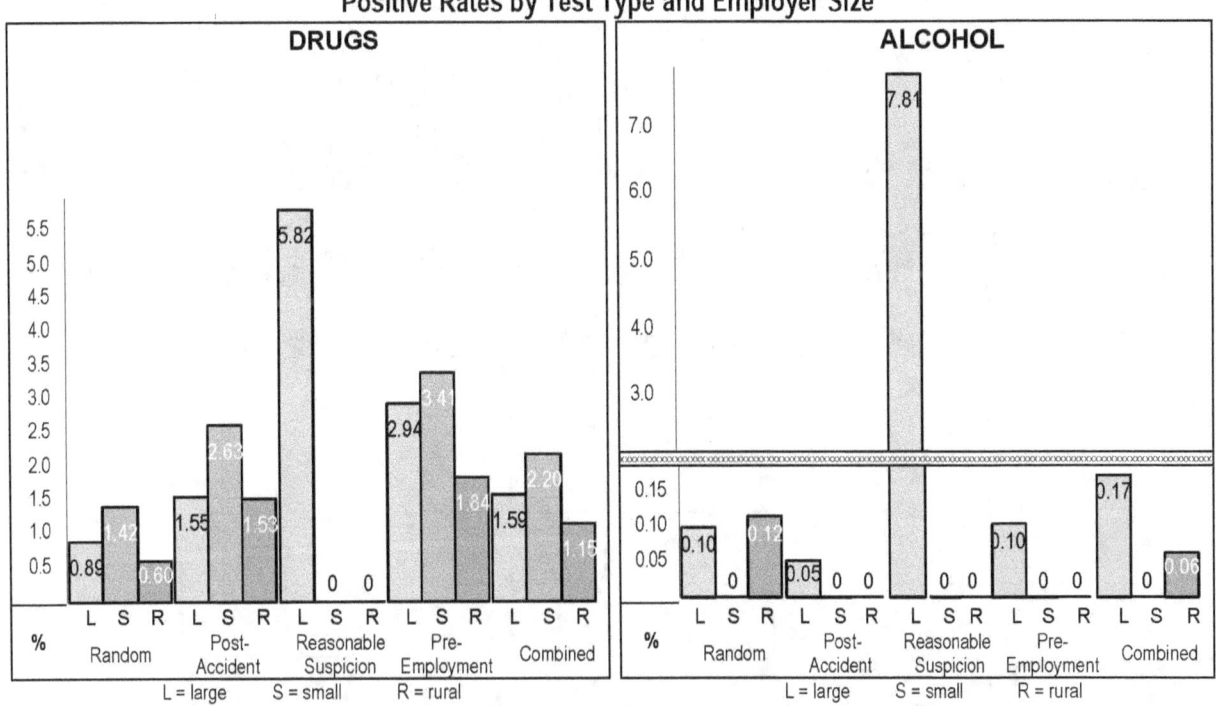

Specimens/Screens Collected and Positives by Test Type and Employer Size

	Drugs						Alcohol					
	Large		Small		Rural		Large		Small		Rural	
	Specimens Collected	Verified Positives	Specimens Collected	Verified Positives	Specimens Collected	Verified Positives	Screens	Confirmed Positives	Screens	Confirmed Positives	Screens	Confirmed Positives
Random	78,831	700	1,195	17	2,487	15	27,015	27	338	0	863	1
Post-Accident	7,850	122	114	3	196	3	7,501	4	100	0	158	0
Reasonable Suspicion	447	26	1	0	4	0	461	36	3	0	5	0
Pre-Employment	40,065	1,177	734	25	1,851	34	8,580	9	29	0	548	0
Total	127,193	2,025	2,044	45	4,538	52	43,557	76	470	0	1,574	1

Note: The graphs subdivided by employer type do not contain columns for employer size that show a positive rate of "0" in the preceding test type/employer size graphs.

Positive Rates by Test Type, Employer Size, and Employer Type

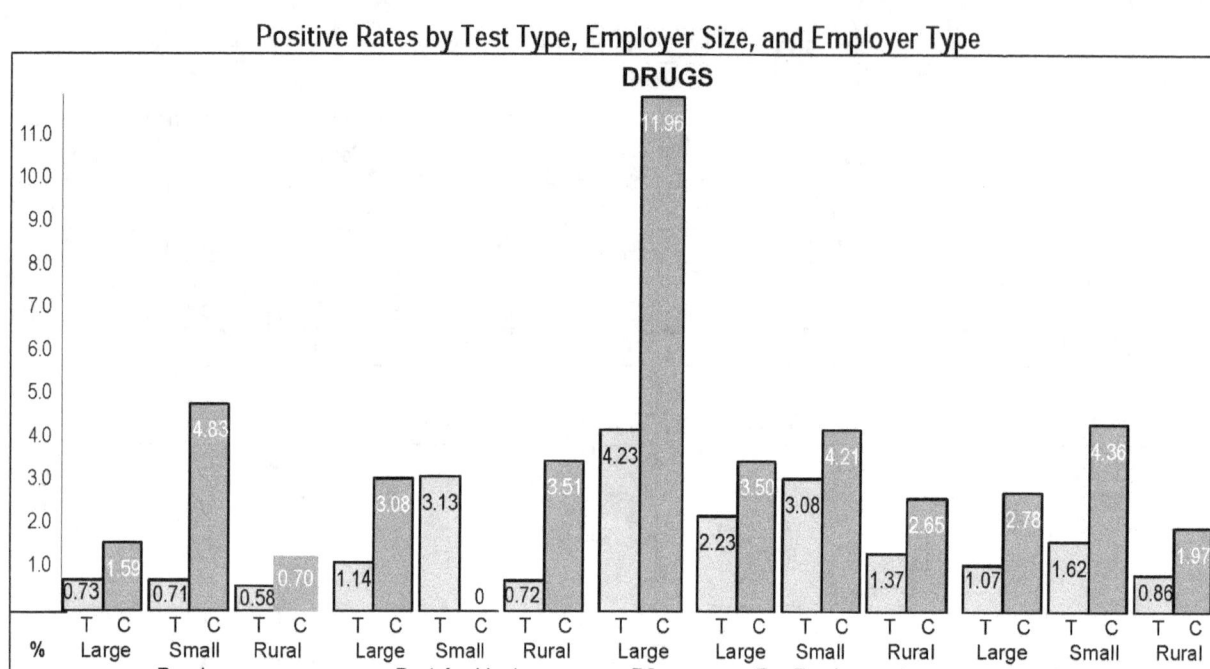

DRUGS

T = transit   C = contractor   RS = Reasonable Suspicion

Positive Rates by Test Type, Employer Size, and Employer Type

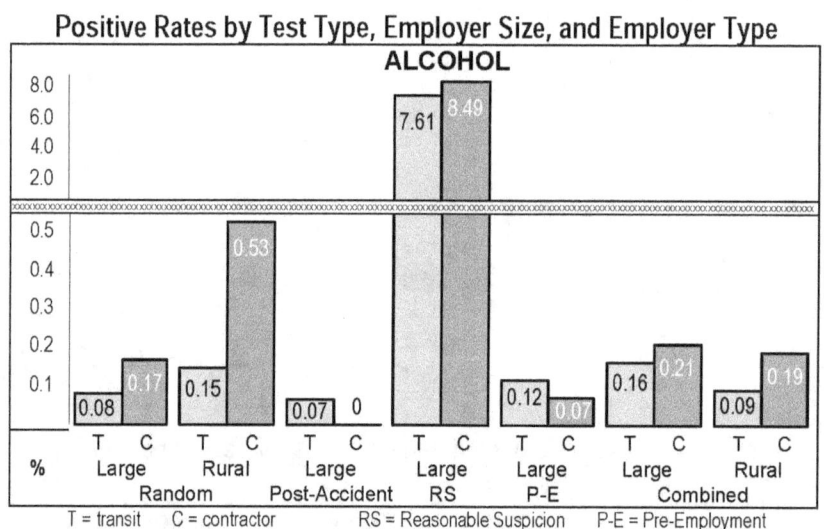

ALCOHOL

T = transit   C = contractor   RS = Reasonable Suspicion   P-E = Pre-Employment

Specimens Collected and Positives by Test Type, Employer Size, and Employer Type

	Drugs											
	Large				Small				Rural			
	Transit		Contractor		Transit		Contractor		Transit		Contractor	
	Specimens Collected	Verified Positives	Specimens Collected	Verified Positives	Specimens Collected	Verified Positives	Specimens Collected	Verified Positives	Specimens Collected	Verified Positives	Specimens Collected	Verified Positives
Random	63,989	464	14,842	236	988	7	207	10	2,059	12	428	3
Post-Accident	6,159	70	1,691	52	96	3	15	0	139	1	57	2
Reasonable Suspicion	355	15	92	11	1	0	0	0	3	0	1	0
Pre-Employment	17,779	396	22,286	781	520	16	214	9	1,172	16	679	18
Total	88,282	945	38,911	1,080	1,605	26	436	19	3,373	29	1,165	23

Screens Collected and Positives by Test Type, Employer Size, and Employer Type

	Alcohol											
	Large				Small				Rural			
	Transit		Contractor		Transit		Contractor		Transit		Contractor	
	Screens	Confirmed Positives	Screens	Confirmed Positives	Screens	Confirmed Positives	Screens	Confirmed Positives	Screens	Confirmed Positives	Screens	Confirmed Positives
Random	22,396	19	4,619	8	290	0	48	0	676	1	187	0
Post-Accident	6,016	4	1,485	0	85	0	15	0	121	0	37	0
Reasonable Suspicion	355	27	106	9	2	0	1	0	3	0	2	0
Pre-Employment	5,873	7	2,707	2	22	0	7	0	254	0	294	0
Total	34,640	57	8,917	19	399	0	71	0	399	1	520	0

3.3.2 Data for Four Test Types by Employee Category

The next two graphs show the positive rates for each test type, as well as the rates for all four types combined, by employee category for drug tests and for alcohol tests, respectively. Two of the reasonable suspicion drug rates are presented on a separate scale because their sample sizes are too small to be considered representative of their populations. Because all of the alcohol rates except reasonable suspicion are 0.2 percent or less, the space below "0.2" in the alcohol graph is expanded under the divider line to allow greater clarity. The table following the graphs provides the statistical basis for the positive rates. These data are further subdivided by employer type and by employer size on the pages that follow.

Positive Rates by Test Type and Employee Category

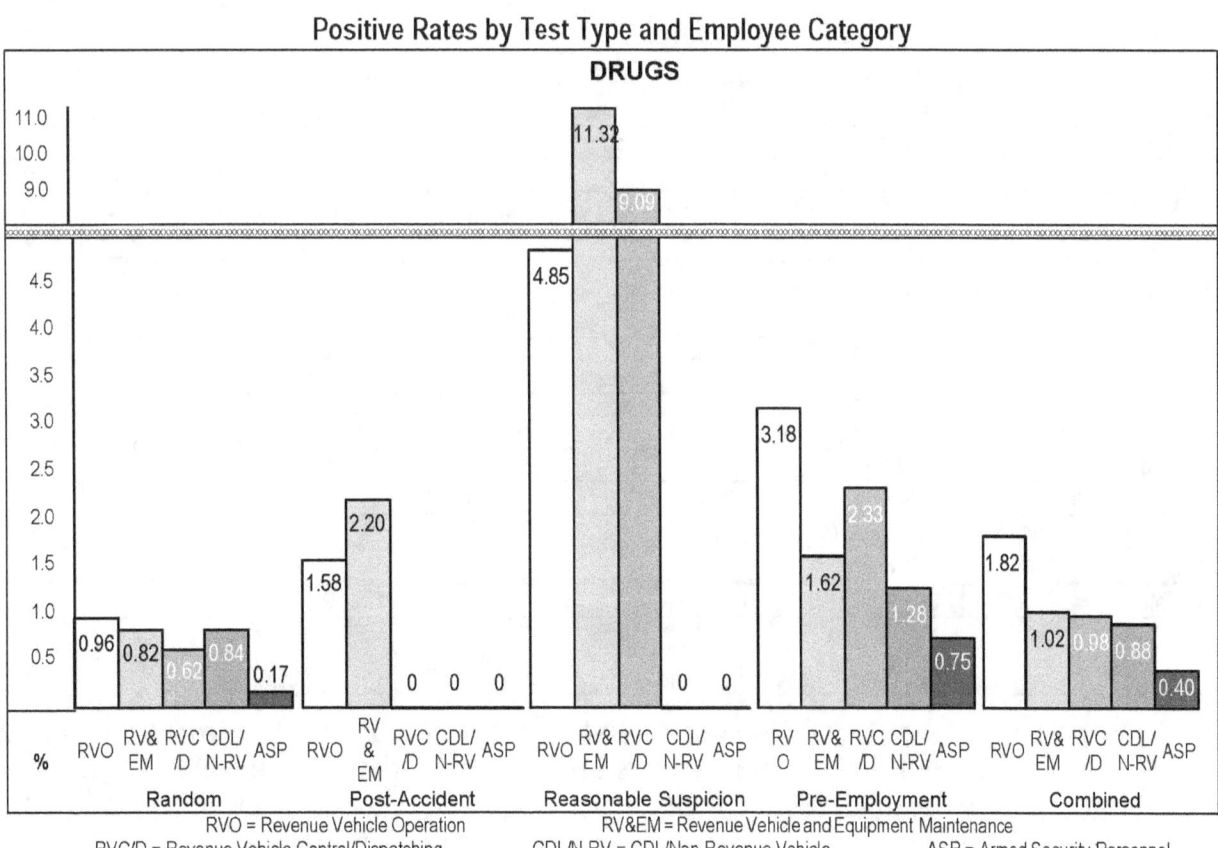

RVO = Revenue Vehicle Operation RV&EM = Revenue Vehicle and Equipment Maintenance
RVC/D = Revenue Vehicle Control/Dispatching CDL/N-RV = CDL/Non-Revenue Vehicle ASP = Armed Security Personnel

Positive Rates by Test Type and Employee Category

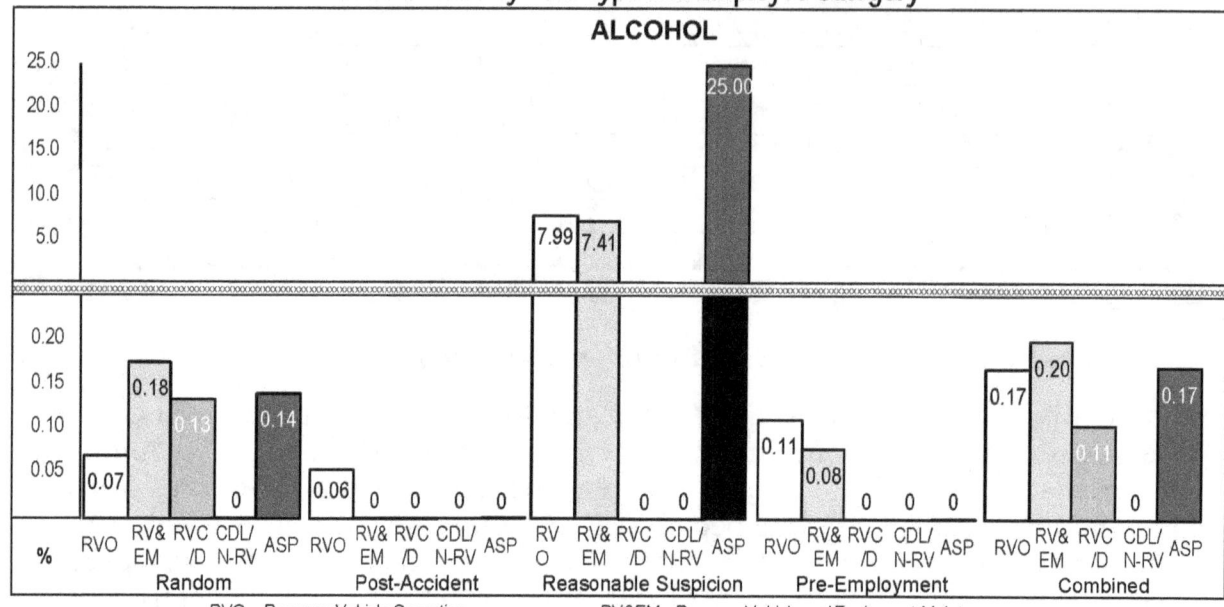

RVO = Revenue Vehicle Operation

RVC/D = Revenue Vehicle Control/Dispatching

RV&EM = Revenue Vehicle and Equipment Maintenance

CDL/N-RV = CDL/Non-Revenue Vehicle

ASP = Armed Security Personnel

Specimens/Screens Collected and Positives by Test Type and Employee Category

	DRUGS									
	Revenue Vehicle Operation		Revenue Vehicle and Equipment Maintenance		Revenue Vehicle Control/Dispatching		CDL/Non-Revenue Vehicle		Armed Security Personnel	
	Specimens Collected	Verified Positives	Specimens Collected	Verified Positives	Specimens Collected	Verified Positives	Specimens Collected	Verified Positives	Specimens Collected	Verified Positives
Random	54,676	525	19,670	161	4,983	31	1,435	12	1,749	3
Post-Accident	7,617	120	363	8	94	0	33	0	53	0
Reasonable Suspicion	371	18	53	6	22	2	1	0	5	0
Pre-Employment	35,152	1,117	4,818	78	1,242	29	235	3	1,203	9
Total	97,816	1,780	24,904	253	6,341	62	1,704	15	3,010	12

	ALCOHOL									
	Revenue Vehicle Operation		Revenue Vehicle and Equipment Maintenance		Revenue Vehicle Control/Dispatching		CDL/Non-Revenue Vehicle		Armed Security Personnel	
	Screens	Confirmed Positives	Screens	Confirmed Positives	Screens	Confirmed Positives	Screens	Confirmed Positives	Screens	Confirmed Positives
Random	18,485	13	6,812	12	1,506	2	696	0	717	1
Post-Accident	7,243	4	342	0	91	0	32	0	51	0
Reasonable Suspicion	388	31	54	4	22	0	1	0	4	1
Pre-Employment	7,152	8	1,278	1	270	0	63	0	394	0
Total	33,268	56	8,486	17	1,889	2	792	0	1,166	2

3.3.2.1 Data for Four Test Types by Employee Category and Employer Type

The following series of graphs subdivide the preceding test type/employee category positive rates by employer type. Two graphs, one for drugs and one for alcohol, are presented for the four test types combined and for each test type. They show the positive rates by employer type for each employee category. This series of graphs is followed by a table that provides the statistical basis for the rates.

Note: The graphs subdivided by employer type do not contain columns for employee categories that show a positive rate of "0" in the preceding test type/employee category graphs.

Positive Rates for Four Test Types Combined by Employee Category and Employer Type

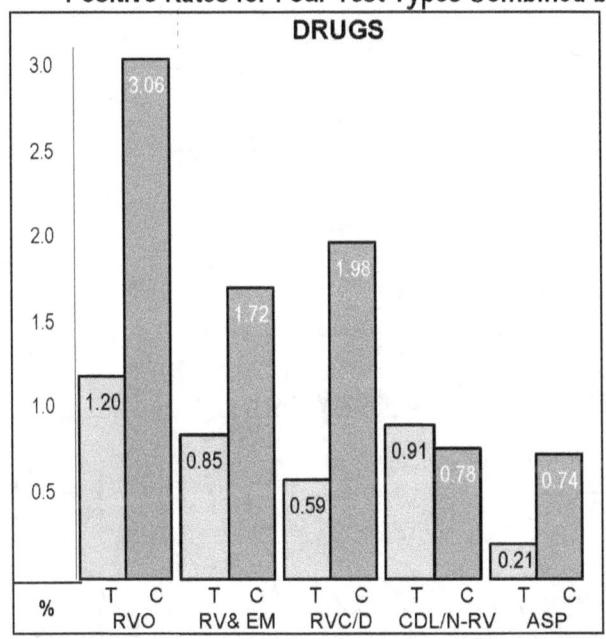

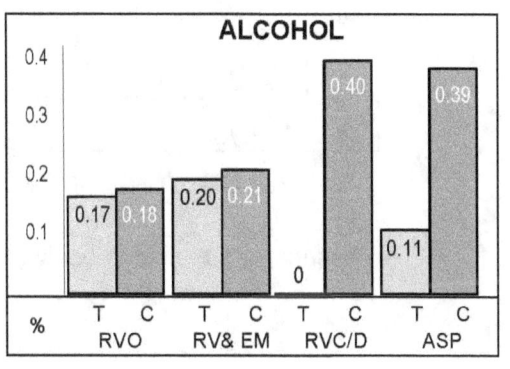

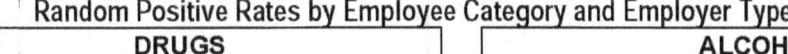

T = transit   C = contractor

RVO = Revenue Vehicle Operation   RV&EM = Revenue Vehicle and Equipment Maintenance

RVC/D = Revenue Vehicle Control/Dispatching   CDL/N-RV = CDL/Non-Revenue Vehicle   ASP = Armed Security Personnel

Random Positive Rates by Employee Category and Employer Type

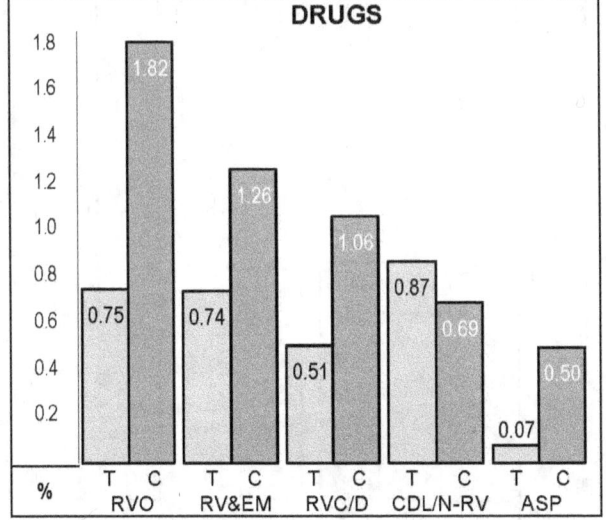

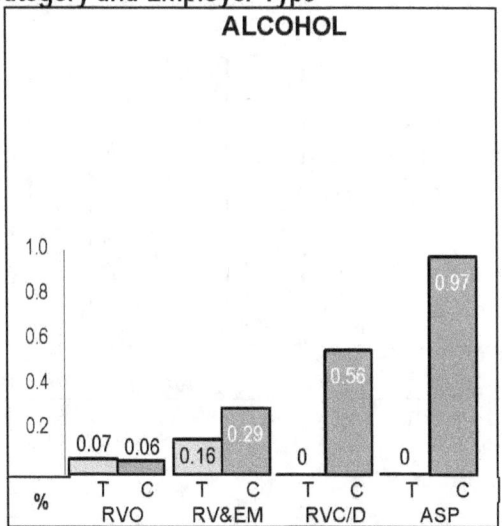

T = transit   C = contractor

RVO = Revenue Vehicle Operation   RV&EM = Revenue Vehicle and Equipment Maintenance

RVC/D = Revenue Vehicle Control/Dispatching   CDL/N-RV = CDL/Non-Revenue Vehicle   ASP = Armed Security Personnel

Post-Accident Positive Rates by Employee Category and Employer Type

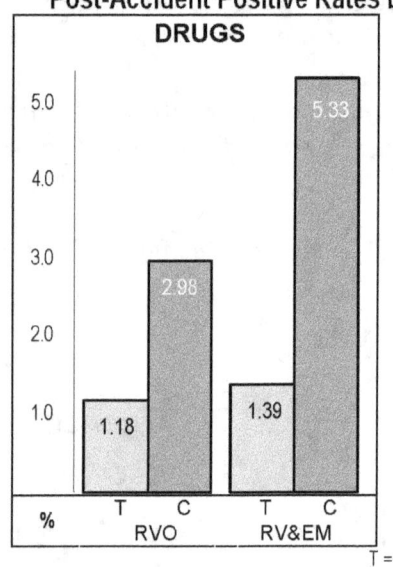

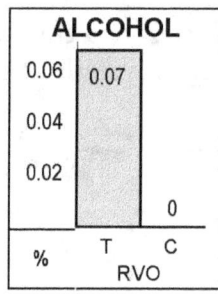

T = transit   C = contractor
RVO = Revenue Vehicle Operation   R&EM = Revenue Vehicle and Equipment Maintenance

Reasonable Suspicion Positive Rates by Employee Category and Employer Type

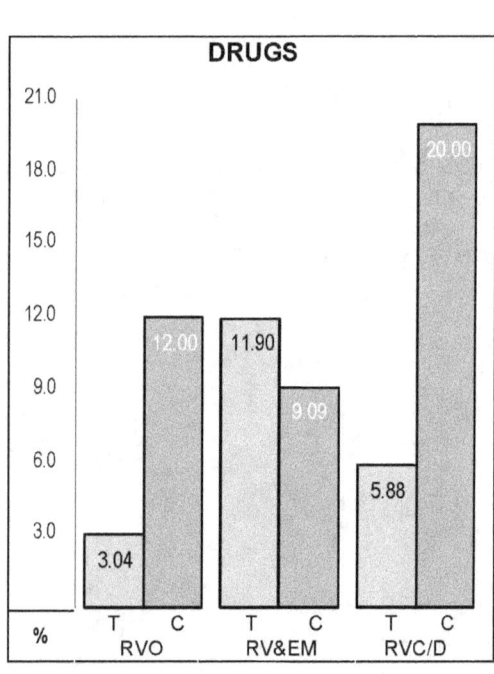

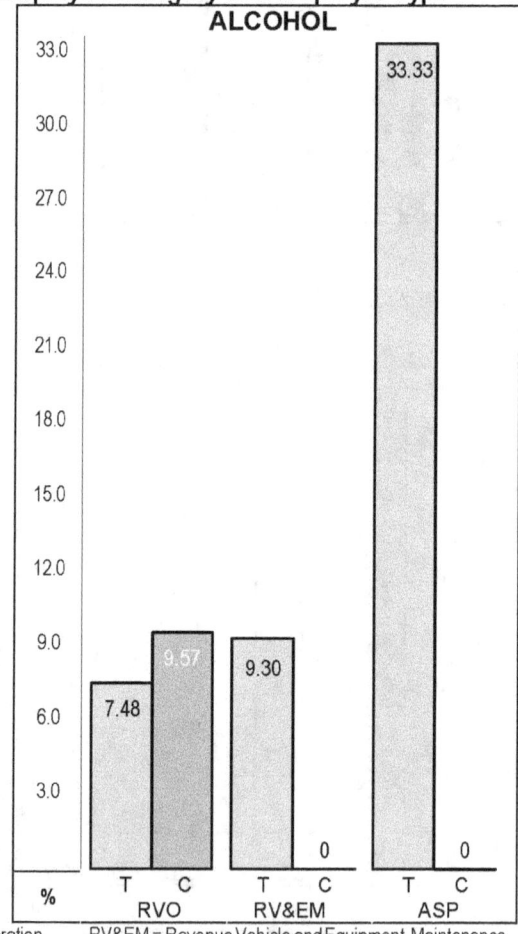

T = transit   C = contractor   RVO = Revenue Vehicle Operation   RV&EM = Revenue Vehicle and Equipment Maintenance
RVC/D = Revenue Vehicle Control/Dispatching   ASP = Armed Security Personnel

Pre-Employment Positive Rates by Employee Category and Employer Type

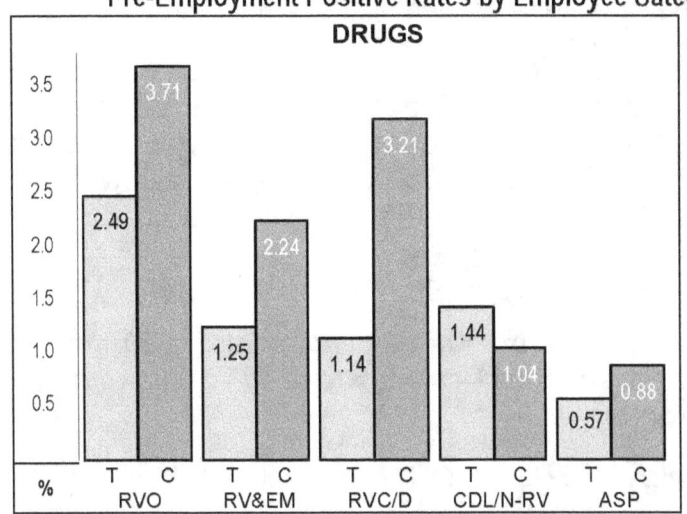

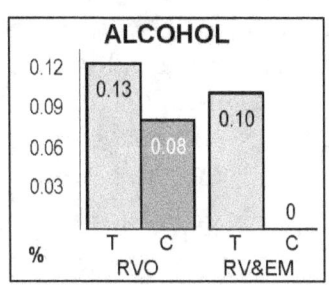

T = transit   C = contractor   RVO = Revenue Vehicle Operation   RV&EM = Revenue Vehicle and Equipment Maintenance
RVC/D = Revenue Vehicle Control/Dispatching   CDL/N-RV = CDL/Non-Revenue Vehicle   ASP = Armed Security Personnel

Specimens/Screens Collected and Positives by Employee Category and Employer Type

		Drugs				Alcohol			
		Transit		Contractor		Transit		Contractor	
		Specimens Collected	Verified Positives	Specimens Collected	Verified Positives	Screens	Confirmed Positives	Screens	Confirmed Positives
Random	RVO	43,781	327	10,895	198	15,183	11	3,302	2
	RV&EM	16,819	125	2,851	36	5,790	9	1,022	3
	RVC/D	3,945	20	1,038	11	1,149	0	357	2
	CDL/N-RV	1,146	10	289	2	626	0	70	0
	ASP	1,345	1	404	2	614	0	103	1
Post-Accident	RVO	5,941	70	1,676	50	5,776	4	1,467	0
	RV&EM	288	4	75	4	282	0	60	0
	RVC/D	84	0	10	0	82	0	9	0
	CDL/N-RV	31	0	2	0	31	0	1	0
	ASP	53	0	0	0	51	0	0	0
Reasonable Suspicion	RVO	296	9	75	9	294	22	94	9
	RV&EM	42	5	11	1	43	4	11	0
	RVC/D	17	1	5	1	19	0	3	0
	CDL/N-RV	1	0	0	0	1	0	0	0
	ASP	3	0	2	0	3	1	1	0
Pre-Employment	RVO	15,250	379	19,902	738	4,760	6	2,392	2
	RV&EM	3,033	38	1,785	40	960	1	318	0
	RVC/D	526	6	716	23	138	0	132	0
	CDL/N-RV	139	2	96	1	52	0	11	0
	ASP	523	3	680	6	239	0	155	0
Total	RVO	65,268	785	32,548	995	26,013	43	7,255	13
	RV&EM	20,182	172	4,722	81	7,075	14	1,411	3
	RVC/D	4,572	27	1,769	35	1,388	0	501	2
	CDL/N-RV	1,317	12	387	3	710	0	82	0
	ASP	1,924	4	1,086	8	907	1	259	1

3.3.2.2 Data for Four Test Types by Employee Category and Employer Size

The following series of graphs subdivide the test type/employee category positive rates by employer size. Two graphs, one for drugs and one for alcohol, are presented for the four test types combined and for each test type. The graphs show the positive rates by employer size for each employee category. However, the alcohol graphs do not contain columns for small employers because no confirmed alcohol positives were reported by small employers. This series of graphs is followed by a table that provides the statistical basis for the rates.

Note: The graphs subdivided by employer size do not contain columns for employee categories that show a positive rate of "0" in the test type/ employee category graphs.

Positive Rates for Four Test Types Combined by Employee Category and Employer Size

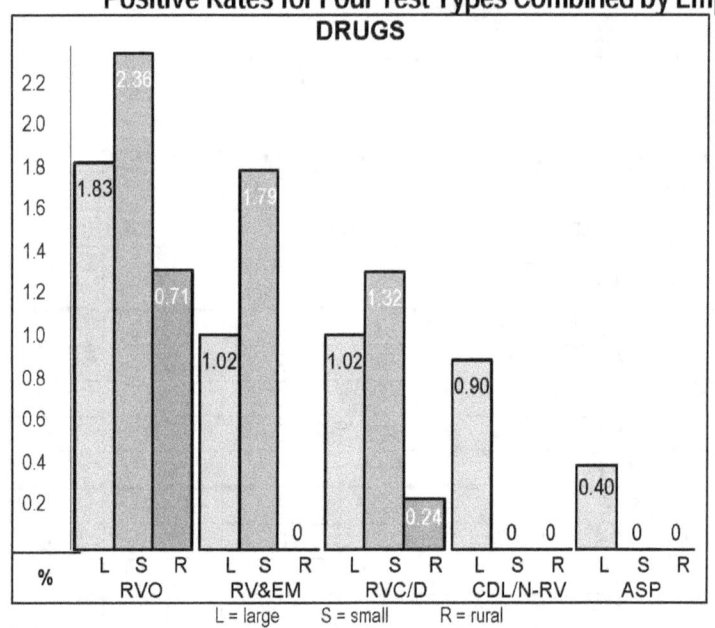

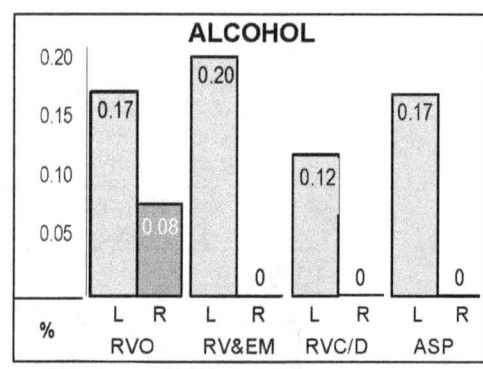

RVO = Revenue Vehicle Operation
RV&EM = Revenue Vehicle and Equipment Maintenance
CDL/N-RV = CDL/Non-Revenue Vehicle
RVC/D = Revenue Vehicle Control/Dispatching
ASP = Armed Security Personnel

Random Positive Rates by Employee Category and Employer Size

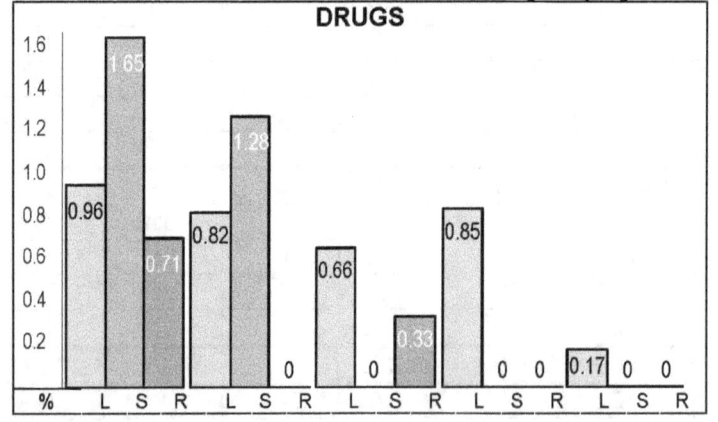

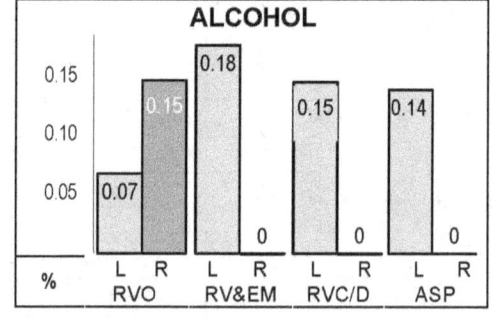

L = large   S = small   R = rural
RVC/D = Revenue Vehicle Control/Dispatching

RVO = Revenue Vehicle Operation
CDL/N-RV = CDL/Non-Revenue Vehicle

RV&EM = Revenue Vehicle and Equipment Maintenance
ASP = Armed Security Personnel

Post-Accident Rates by Employee Category and Employer Size

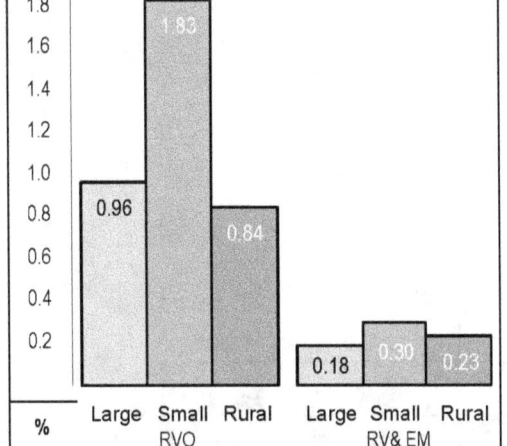

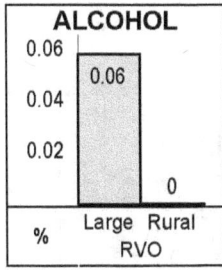

RVO = Revenue Vehicle Operation
RV&EM = Revenue Vehicle and Equipment Maintenance

One of the rates in the next alcohol graph is presented on a separate scale because its sample size is too small to be representative of its population.

Reasonable Suspicion Rates by Employee Category and Employer Size

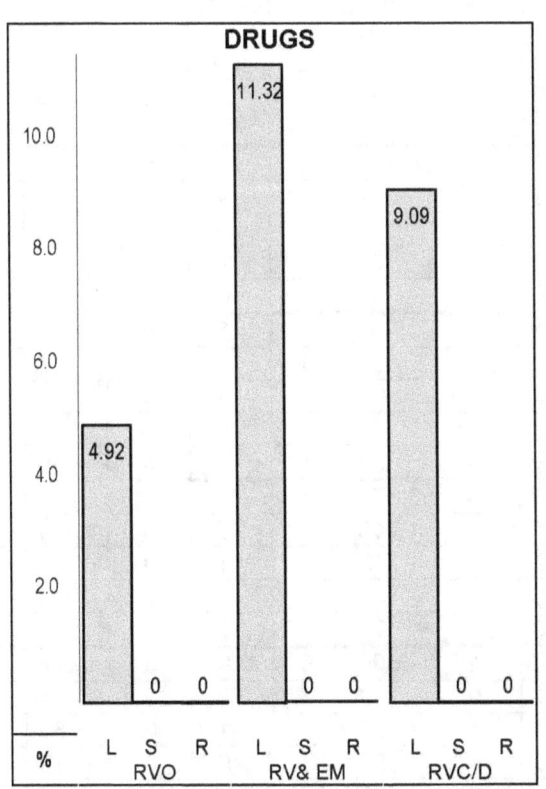

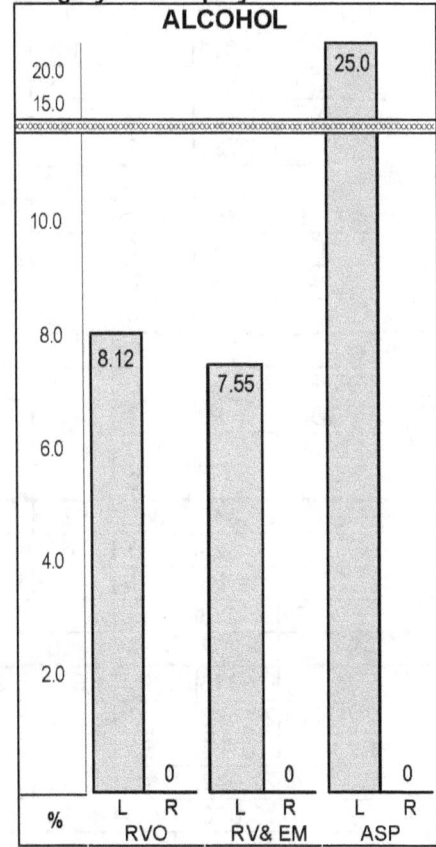

L = large   S = small   R = rural
RV&EM = Revenue Vehicle and Equipment Maintenance   RVC/D = Revenue Vehicle Control/Dispatching   ASP = Armed Security Personnel

RVO = Revenue Vehicle Operation

Pre-Employment Rates by Employee Category and Employer Size

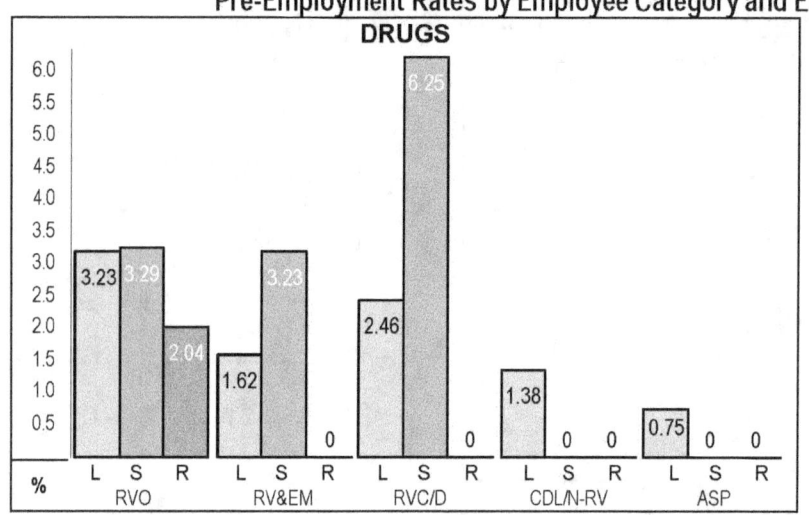

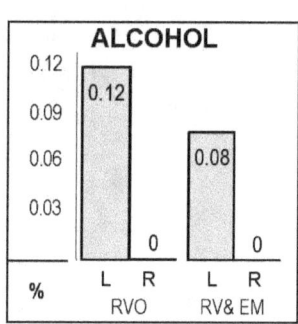

L = large   S = small   R = rural   RVO = Revenue Vehicle Operation   RV&EM = Revenue Vehicle and Equipment Maintenance
RVC/D = Revenue Vehicle Control/Dispatching   CDL/N-RV = CDL/Non-Revenue Vehicle   ASP = Armed Security Personnel

Specimens/Screens Collected and Positives by Employee Category and Employer Size

| | | Drugs | | | | | | Alcohol | | | | | |
| | | Large | | Small | | Rural | | Large | | Small | | Rural | |
		Specimens Collected	Verified Positives	Specimens Collected	Verified Positives	Specimens Collected	Verified Positives	Screens	Confirmed Positives	Screens	Confirmed Positives	Screens	Confirmed Positives
Random	RVO	51,784	496	907	15	1,985	14	17,550	12	264	0	671	1
	RV&EM	19,331	159	156	2	183	0	6,701	12	43	0	68	0
	RVC/D	4,561	30	119	0	303	1	1,359	2	29	0	118	0
	CDL/N-RV	1,416	12	3	0	16	0	690	0	0	0	6	0
	ASP	1,739	3	10	0	0	0	715	1	2	0	0	0
Post-Accident	RVO	7,318	114	108	3	191	3	6,997	4	96	0	150	0
	RV&EM	358	8	5	0	0	0	337	0	4	0	1	0
	RVC/D	89	0	1	0	4	0	86	0	0	0	5	0
	CDL/N-RV	32	0	0	0	1	0	30	0	0	0	2	0
	ASP	53	0	0	0	0	0	51	0	0	0	0	0
Reasonable Suspicion	RVO	366	18	1	0	4	0	382	31	2	0	4	0
	RV&EM	53	6	0	0	0	0	53	4	0	0	1	0
	RVC/D	22	2	0	0	0	0	21	0	1	0	0	0
	CDL/N-RV	1	0	0	0	0	0	1	0	0	0	0	0
	ASP	5	0	0	0	0	0	4	1	0	0	0	0
Pre-Employment	RVO	32,848	1,062	639	21	1,665	34	6,671	8	22	0	459	0
	RV&EM	4,698	76	62	2	58	0	1,248	1	6	0	24	0
	RVC/D	1,098	27	32	2	112	0	212	0	1	0	57	0
	CDL/N-RV	218	3	1	0	16	0	55	0	0	0	8	0
	ASP	1,203	9	0	0	0	0	394	0	0	0	0	0
Total	RVO	92,316	1,690	1,655	39	3,845	51	31,600	55	384	0	1,284	1
	RV&EM	24,440	249	223	4	241	0	8,339	17	53	0	94	0
	RVC/D	5,770	59	152	2	419	1	1,678	2	31	0	180	0
	CDL/N-RV	1,667	15	4	0	33	0	776	0	0	0	16	0
	ASP	3,000	12	10	0	0	0	31,600	55	384	0	1,284	1

3.3.3 Data for Four Test Types by FTA Region

The following two maps show the positive rates for all four test types combined for drugs and for alcohol for each of FTA's ten regions. The shading variations provide quick comparison. The exact rates are also included. The statistical basis for those rates is provided in the accompanying tables.

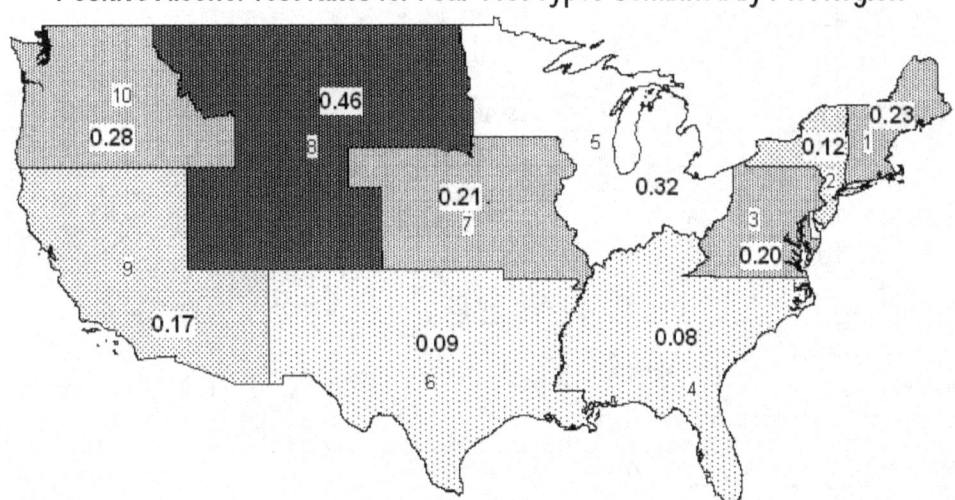

Positive Drug Test Rates for Four Test Types Combined by FTA Region

Specimens Collected and Positives by Region

Region	Specimens Collected	Verified Positives
1	4,438	48
2	34,385	437
3	18,780	451
4	13,304	164
5	19,392	334
6	9,361	130
7	1,774	19
8	5,667	96
9	18,332	372
10	8,342	71

Positive Alcohol Test Rates for Four Test Types Combined by FTA Region

Screens Collected and Positives by Region

Region	Screens	Confirmed Positives
1	877	2
2	11,235	13
3	9,216	18
4	6,538	5
5	4,690	15
6	4,412	4
7	483	1
8	875	4
9	4,759	8
10	2,516	7

These data are subdivided by employer type and by employer size on the following pages. The drug positive rates by employer type, the drug positive rates for large employers, and the alcohol positive rates for large employers are displayed on maps. The statistical basis for the rates is provided in the accompanying tables. Because of the low number of positives reported for the other categories (alcohol by employer type and small and rural employers), the rates for those categories appear in tables, along with the statistical basis for those rates.

Positive Drug Test Rates for Four Test Types Combined by FTA Region and Employer Type

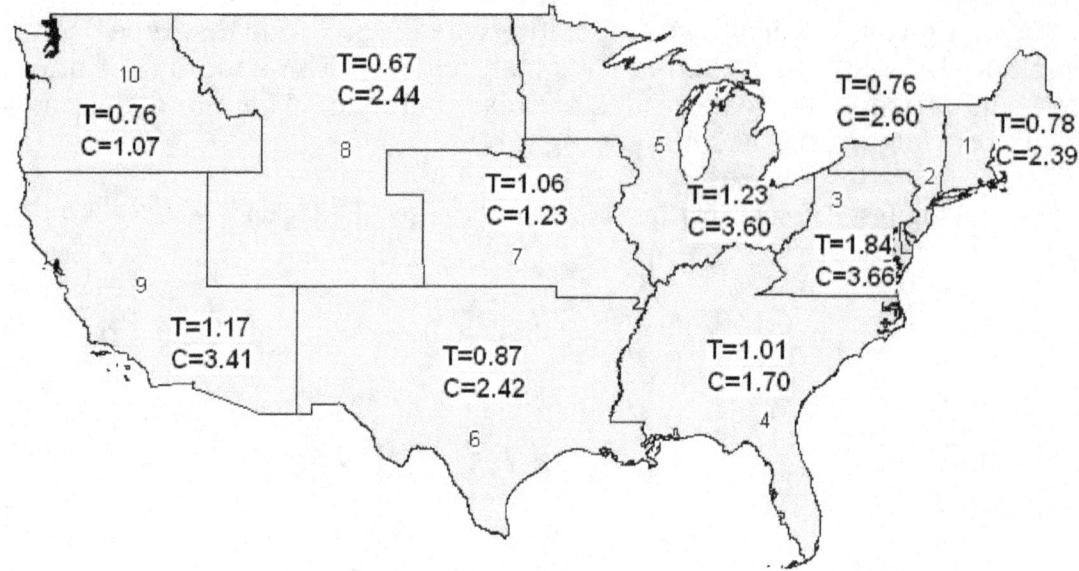

Drug Specimens Collected and Verified Positives by Region and Employer Type

Region	Transit		Contractor	
	Specimens Collected	Verified Positives	Specimens Collected	Verified Positives
1	3,602	28	836	20
2	24,855	189	9,530	248
3	12,995	239	5,785	212
4	9,013	91	4,291	73
5	15,341	188	4,051	146
6	6,221	54	3,140	76
7	1,611	17	163	2
8	2,384	16	3,283	80
9	11,326	133	7,006	239
10	5,915	45	2,427	26

Alcohol Data for Four Test Types Combined by Region and Employer Type

Region	Transit			Contractor		
	Screens	Confirmed Positives	Positive Rate	Screens	Confirmed Positives	Positive Rate
1	746	2	0.27	131	0	0.00
2	8,527	8	0.09	2,708	5	0.18
3	7,031	14	0.20	2,185	4	0.18
4	5,112	4	0.08	1,426	1	0.07
5	3,835	14	0.37	855	1	0.12
6	3,739	4	0.11	673	0	0.00
7	479	1	0.21	4	0	0.00
8	533	1	0.19	342	3	0.88
9	4,034	6	0.15	725	2	0.28
10	2,057	4	0.19	459	3	0.65

Positive Drug Test Rates for Four Test Types Combined by FTA Region and Employer Size—Large

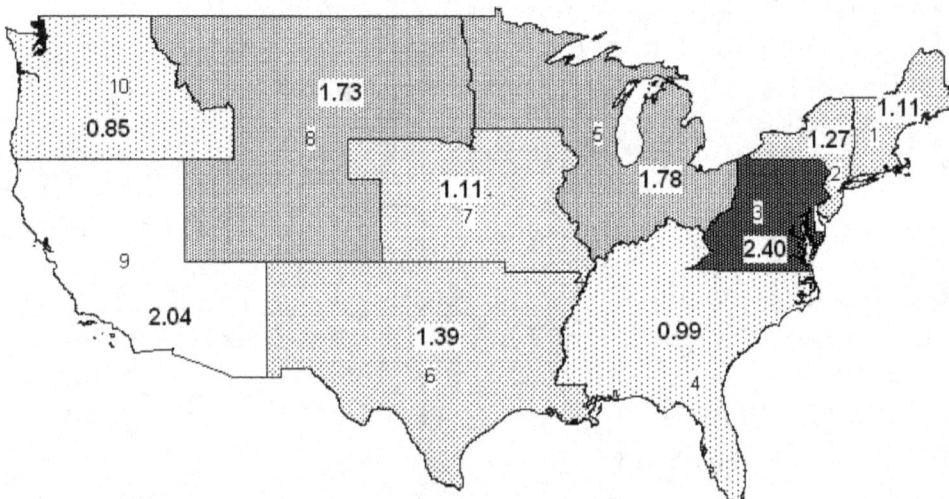

Specimens Collected & Positives by Region and Large Employers

Region	Specimens Collected	Verified Positives
1	4,313	48
2	34,385	437
3	18,780	451
4	10,155	101
5	17,588	313
6	9,240	128
7	1,705	19
8	5,534	96
9	18,076	369
10	7,417	63

Positive Alcohol Test Rates for Four Test Types Combined by FTA Region and Employer Size—Large

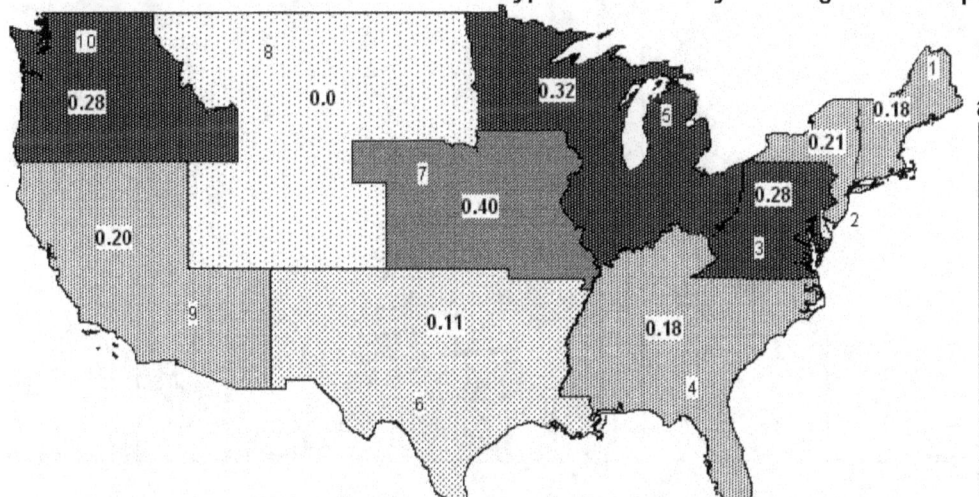

Screens Collected & Positives by Region and Large Employers

Region	Screens	Confirmed Positives
1	850	2
2	11,235	13
3	9,216	18
4	5,432	5
5	4,242	15
6	4,353	4
7	468	1
8	834	4
9	4,727	8
10	2,200	6

Data for Four Test Types Combined by FTA Region and Employer Size—Small and Rural

	Drugs						Alcohol					
	Small			Rural			Small			Rural		
Region	Specimens Collected	Verified Positives	Positive Rate	Specimens Collected	Verified Positives	Positive Rate	Screens	Confirmed Positives	Positive Rate	Screens	Confirmed Positives	Positive Rate
1	125	0	0	0	0	0	27	0	0	0	0	0
2	0	0	0	0	0	0	0	0	0	0	0	0
3	0	0	0	0	0	0	0	0	0	0	0	0
4	717	28	3.91%	2,432	0.85%	10	155	0	0	951	0	0
5	623	12	1.93%	1,181	0.55%	4	141	0	0	307	0	0
6	121	2	1.65%	0	0	0	59	0	0	0	0	0
7	69	0	0	0	0	0	15	0	0	0	0	0
8	133	0	0	0	0	0	41	0	0	0	0	0
9	256	3	1.17%	0	0	0	32	0	0	0	0	0
10	0	0	0	925	1.18%	7	0	0	0	316	1	0.32%

The data for calculating the verified positive rates by region for random tests alone appear in the tables of regional random test violation data, in Section 3.1.2. Regional data for the other three test types are insufficient to calculate meaningful rates or to accurately normalize the data reported.

3.4 Test Data by Type of Drug

The verified positive rates[6] for each type of drug tested for are presented for each test type and for the four test types combined in the following graph. A table follows that provides the statistical basis for the positive rates. The table is followed by charts that show the percentage by drug type of the total drug type detections[7] for each test type and the four types combined. These rates and data are presented by employer type, employer size, and employee category later in this section.

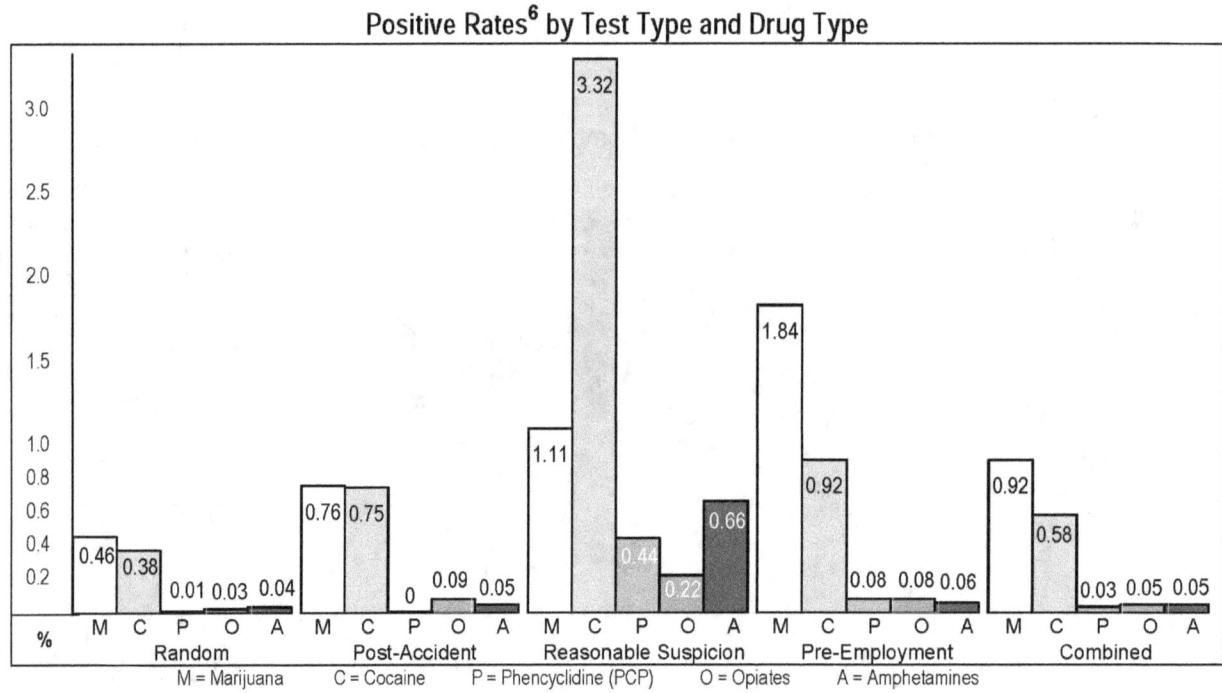

Positive Rates[6] by Test Type and Drug Type

M = Marijuana   C = Cocaine   P = Phencyclidine (PCP)   O = Opiates   A = Amphetamines

Specimens Collected and Positives by Test Type and Drug Type

	Specimens Collected	Verified Positives				
		Marijuana	Cocaine	PCP	Opiates	Amphetamines
Random	82,513	378	313	8	23	30
Post-Accident	8,160	62	61	0	7	4
Reasonable Suspicion	452	5	15	2	1	3
Pre-Employment	42,650	785	392	35	33	26
Total	133,775	1,230	781	45	64	63

---

[6] For clarity in presenting the test results, "positive rate" is used differently in this report than in Part 655. Here, it does not include refusals. See the text box in Section 2.3 for a full explanation.

[7] Because multiple drugs are sometimes detected in one specimen, the total number of drug detections may be greater than the total number of verified positives.

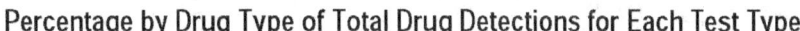

Percentage by Drug Type of Total Drug Detections for Each Test Type

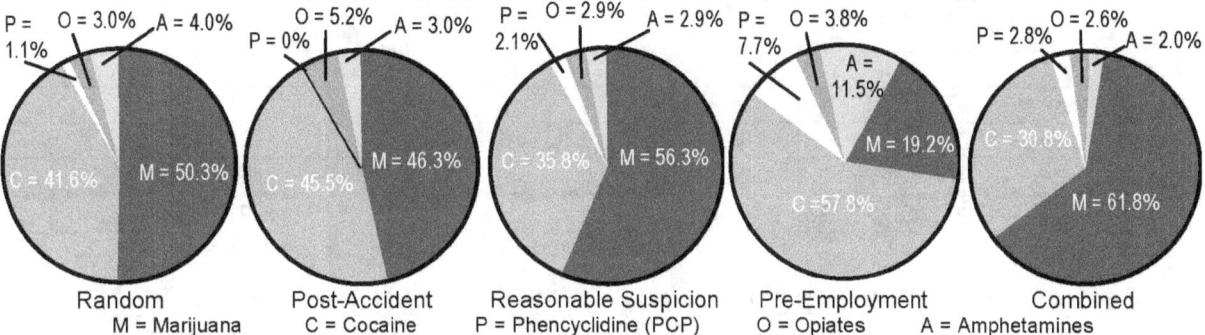

| Random | Post-Accident | Reasonable Suspicion | Pre-Employment | Combined |

P = Phencyclidine (PCP)

M = Marijuana   C = Cocaine   P = Phencyclidine (PCP)   O = Opiates   A = Amphetamines

3.4.1 Data by Test Type, Employer Type, and Drug Type

The following three graphs show the positive rates by drug type for each test type and for the four test types combined by employer type. Two different scales are used in the reasonable suspicion graph to accommodate the disparity in rates. Two tables follow the graphs. The first provides the statistical basis for the rates. The second shows the percentage by drug type of the total drug type detections for each test type and the four test types combined by employer type.

Positive Rates by Test Type, Employer Type, and Drug Type

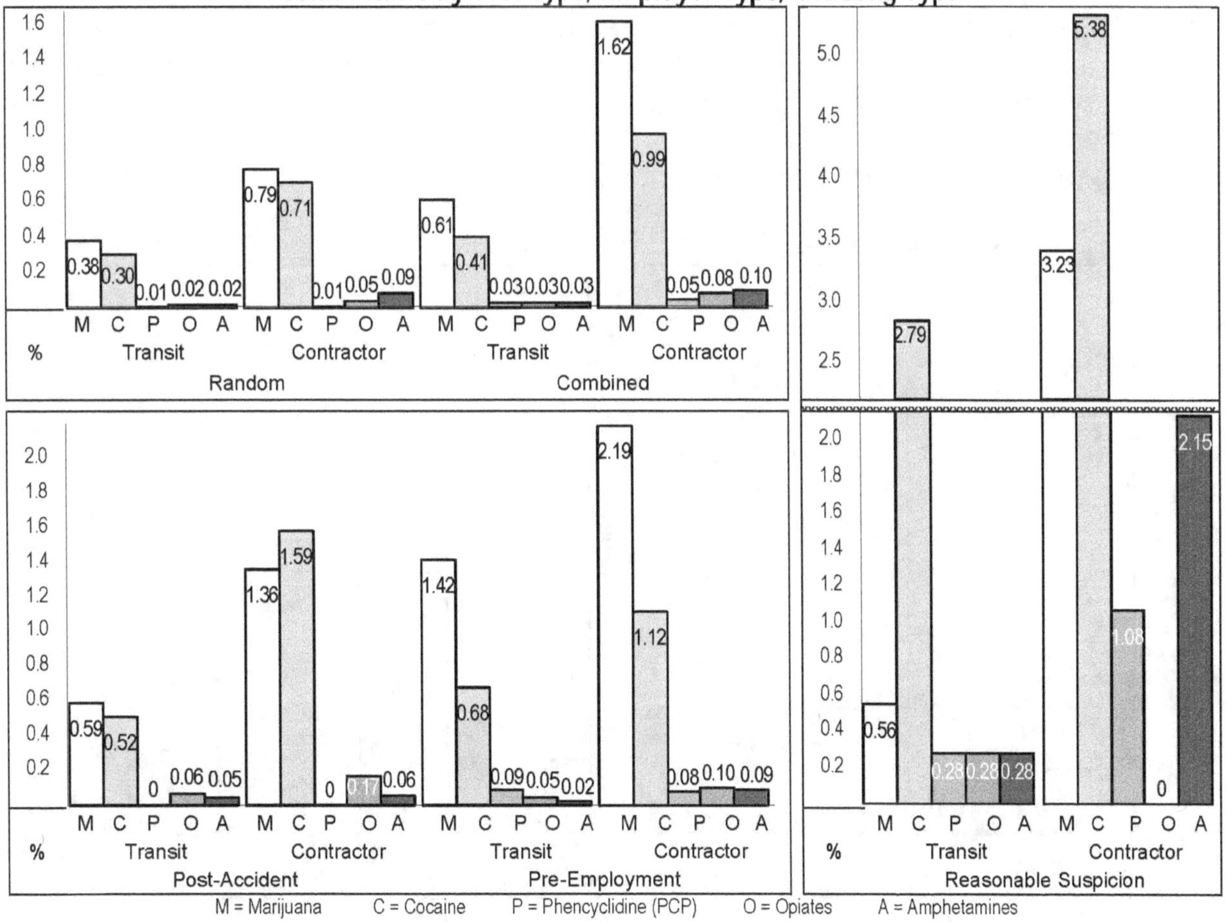

M = Marijuana   C = Cocaine   P = Phencyclidine (PCP)   O = Opiates   A = Amphetamines

Specimens Collected and Positives by Test Type, Employer Size, and Drug Type

	Transit						Contractor					
	SC	M	C	P	O	A	SC	M	C	P	O	A
Random	67,036	255	203	7	16	16	15,477	123	110	1	7	14
Post-Accident	6,397	38	33	0	4	3	1,763	24	28	0	3	1
Reasonable Suspicion	359	2	10	1	1	1	93	3	5	1	0	2
Pre-Employment	19,471	277	133	17	9	4	23,179	508	259	18	24	22
Total	93,263	572	379	25	30	24	40,512	658	402	20	34	39

SC = specimens collected   M = Marijuana   C = Cocaine   P = Phencyclidine (PCP)   O = Opiates   A = Amphetamines

Percentage by Drug Type of Total Drug Detections for Each Test Type by Employer Type

	Transit					Contractor				
	Marijuana	Cocaine	PCP	Opiates	Amphetamines	Marijuana	Cocaine	PCP	Opiates	Amphetamines
Random	51.3	40.9	1.4	3.2	3.2	48.2	43.1	0.4	2.8	5.5
Post-Accident	48.7	42.3	0	5.1	3.9	42.8	50.0	0	5.4	1.8
Reasonable Suspicion	13.3	66.6	6.7	6.7	6.7	27.3	45.4	9.1	0	18.2
Pre-Employment	63.0	30.2	3.9	2.0	0.9	61.1	31.2	2.2	2.9	2.6
Combined	55.6	36.8	2.4	2.9	2.3	57.1	34.9	1.7	2.9	3.4

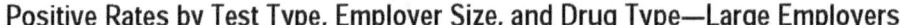

3.4.2 Data by Test Type, Employer Size, and Drug Type

The following four graphs show the rates by drug type for each test type and for the four test types combined by employer size--the first graph for large employers and the other three for small and rural. Two tables follow the graphs. The first provides the statistical basis for the rates. The second shows the percentage by drug type of the total drug type detections for each test type by employer size.

Positive Rates by Test Type, Employer Size, and Drug Type—Large Employers

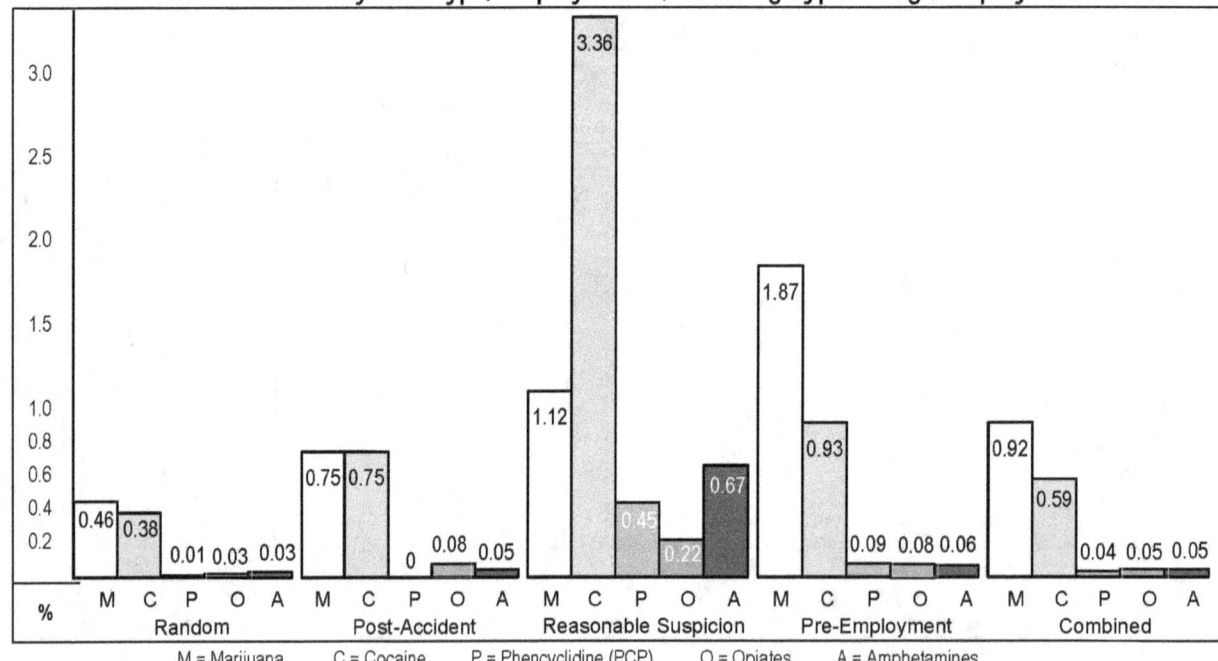

M = Marijuana   C = Cocaine   P = Phencyclidine (PCP)   O = Opiates   A = Amphetamines

Positive Rates by Test Type, Employer Size, and Drug Type—Small and Rural Employers

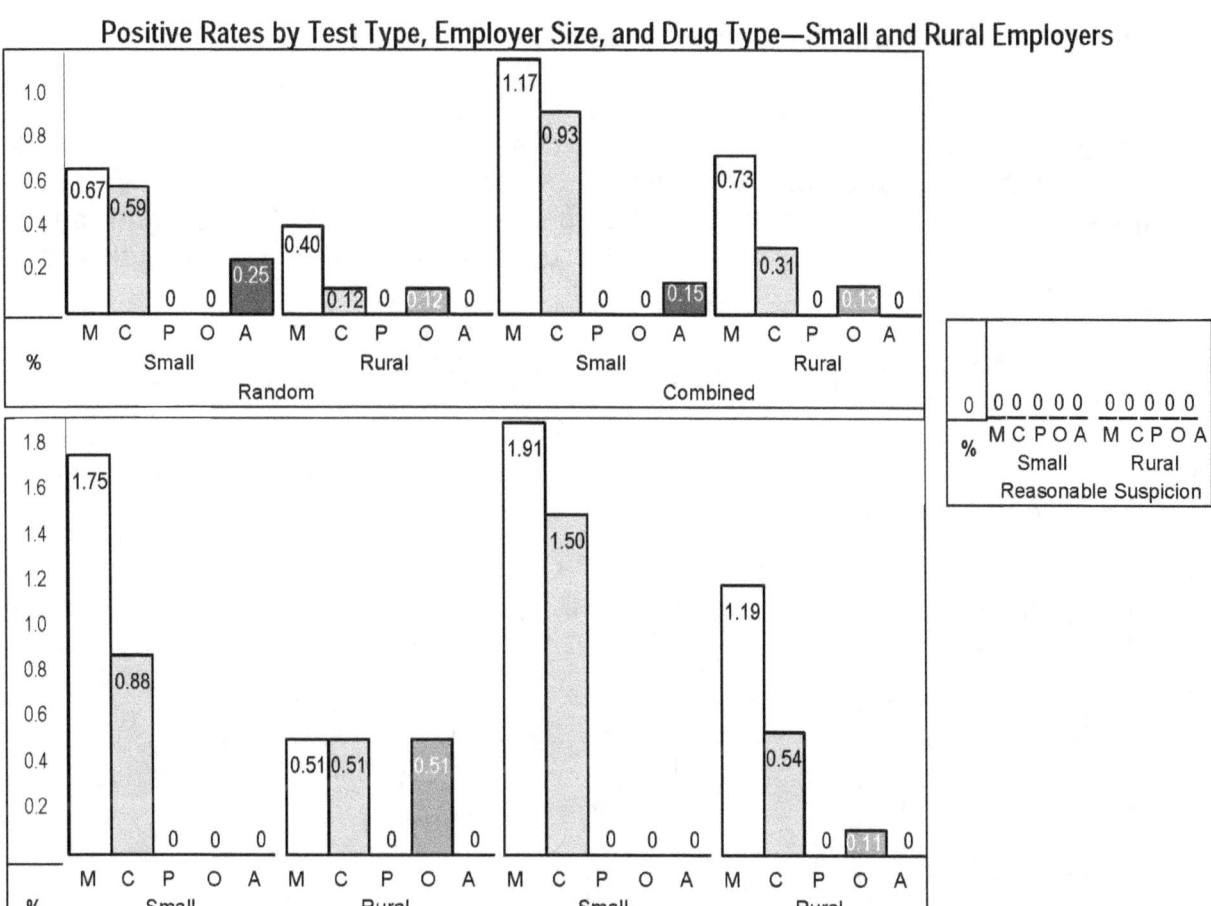

S = small   R = rural   M = Marijuana   C = Cocaine   P = Phencyclidine (PCP)   O = Opiates   A = Amphetamines

Specimens Collected and Positives by Test Type, Employer Size, and Drug Type

	Large						Small						Rural					
	SC	M	C	P	O	A	SC	M	C	P	O	A	SC	M	C	P	O	A
Random	78,831	360	303	8	20	27	1,195	8	8	0	0	3	2,487	10	3	0	3	0
Post-Accident	7,850	59	59	0	6	4	114	2	2	0	0	0	196	1	1	0	1	0
Reasonable Suspicion	447	5	15	2	1	3	1	0	0	0	0	0	4	0	0	0	0	0
Pre-Employment	40,065	749	371	35	31	26	734	14	14	0	0	0	1,851	22	10	0	2	0
Total	127,193	1,173	748	45	58	60	2,044	24	24	0	0	3	4,538	33	14	0	6	0

SC = specimens collected   M = Marijuana   C = Cocaine   P = Phencyclidine (PCP)   O = Opiates   A = Amphetamines

Percentage by Drug Type of Total Drug Detections for Each Test Type by Employer Size

	Large					Small					Rural				
	M	C	P	O	A	M	C	P	O	A	M	C	P	O	A
Random	50.1	42.2	1.1	2.8	3.8	44.4	38.9	0	0	16.7	62.5	18.75	0	18.75	0
Post-Accident	46.1	46.1	0	4.7	3.1	66.7	33.3	0	0	0	33.3	33.3	0	33.3	0
Reasonable Suspicion	19.2	57.7	7.7	3.9	11.5	0	0	0	0	0	0	0	0	0	0
Pre-Employment	61.8	30.6	2.9	2.6	2.1	56.0	44.0	0	0	0	64.7	29.4	0	5.9	0
Combined	56.3	35.9	2.2	2.8	2.9	52.2	41.3	0	0	6.5	62.3	26.4	0	11.3	0

M = Marijuana   C = Cocaine   P = Phencyclidine (PCP)   O = Opiates   A = Amphetamines

3.4.3 Data by Test Type, Employee Category, and Drug Type

The following five graphs show the rates by drug type for each test type and for the four test types combined by employee category. A graph is presented for the four test types combined and for each of the test types. Two tables follow the graphs. The first provides the statistical basis for the rates. The second shows the percentage by drug type of the total drug type detections for each test type and the four test types combined by employee category.

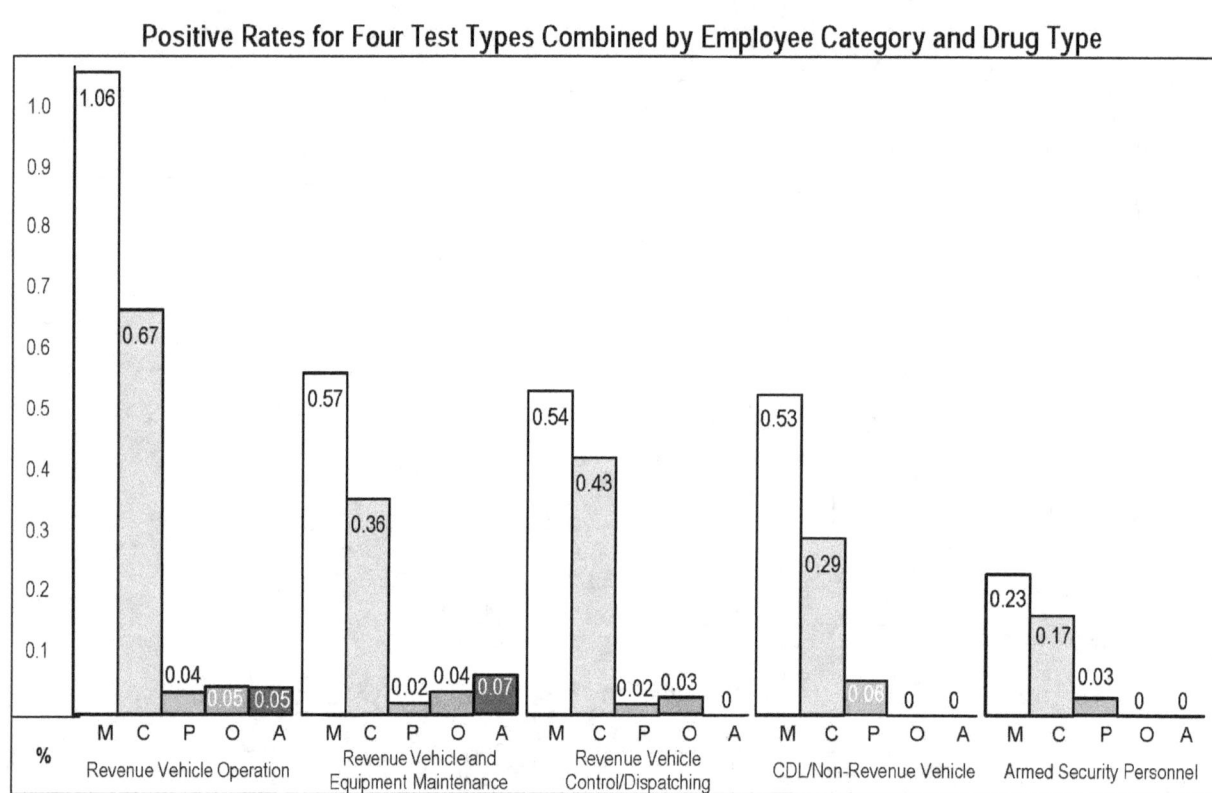

Positive Rates for Four Test Types Combined by Employee Category and Drug Type

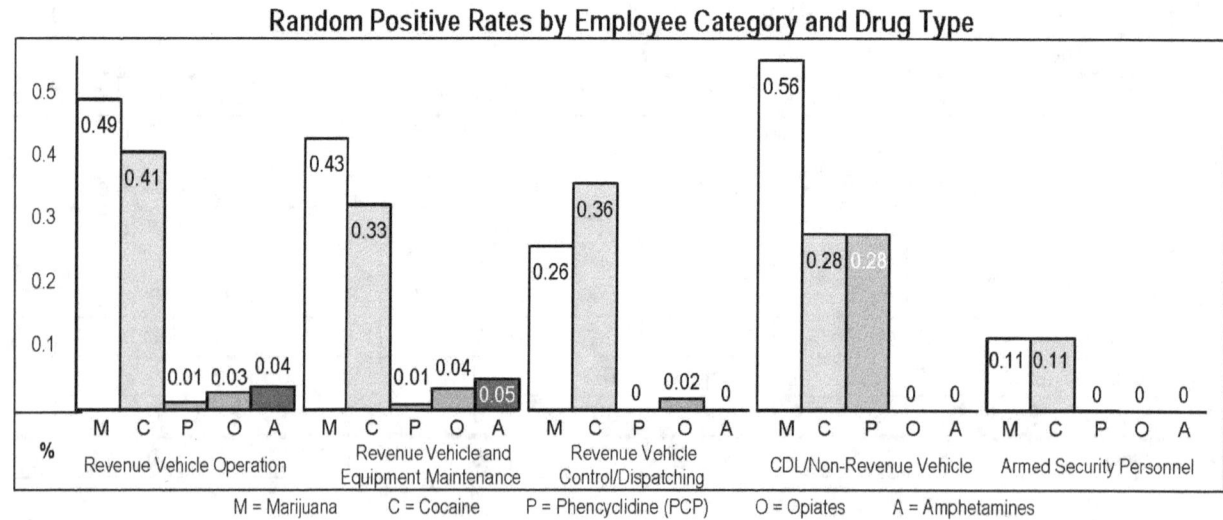

Random Positive Rates by Employee Category and Drug Type

Post-Accident Positive Rates by Employee Category and Drug Type

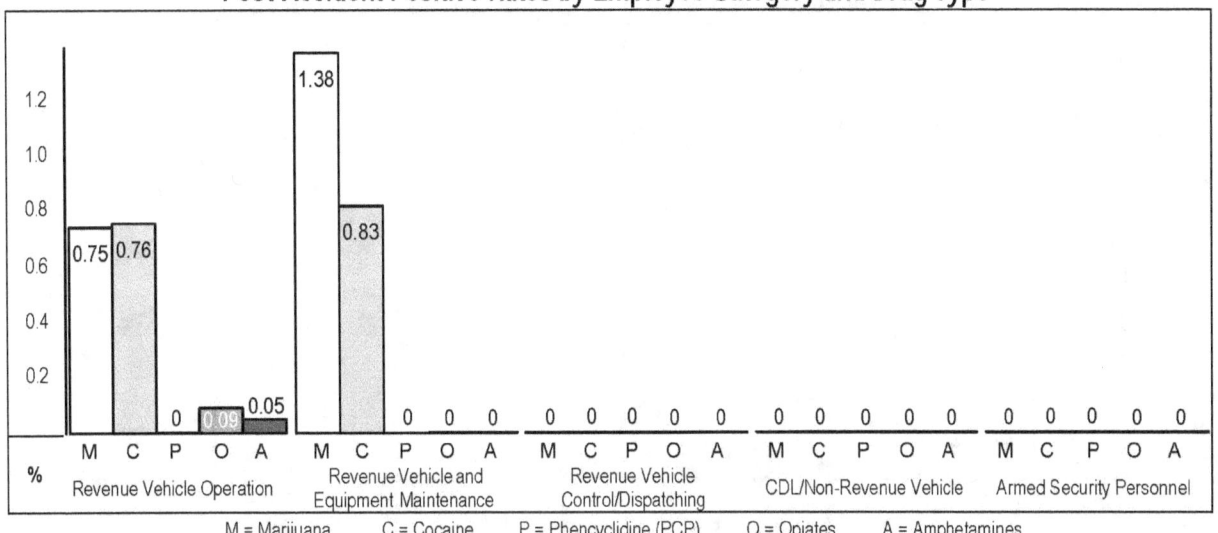

M = Marijuana   C = Cocaine   P = Phencyclidine (PCP)   O = Opiates   A = Amphetamines

Reasonable Suspicion Positive Rates by Employee Category and Drug Type

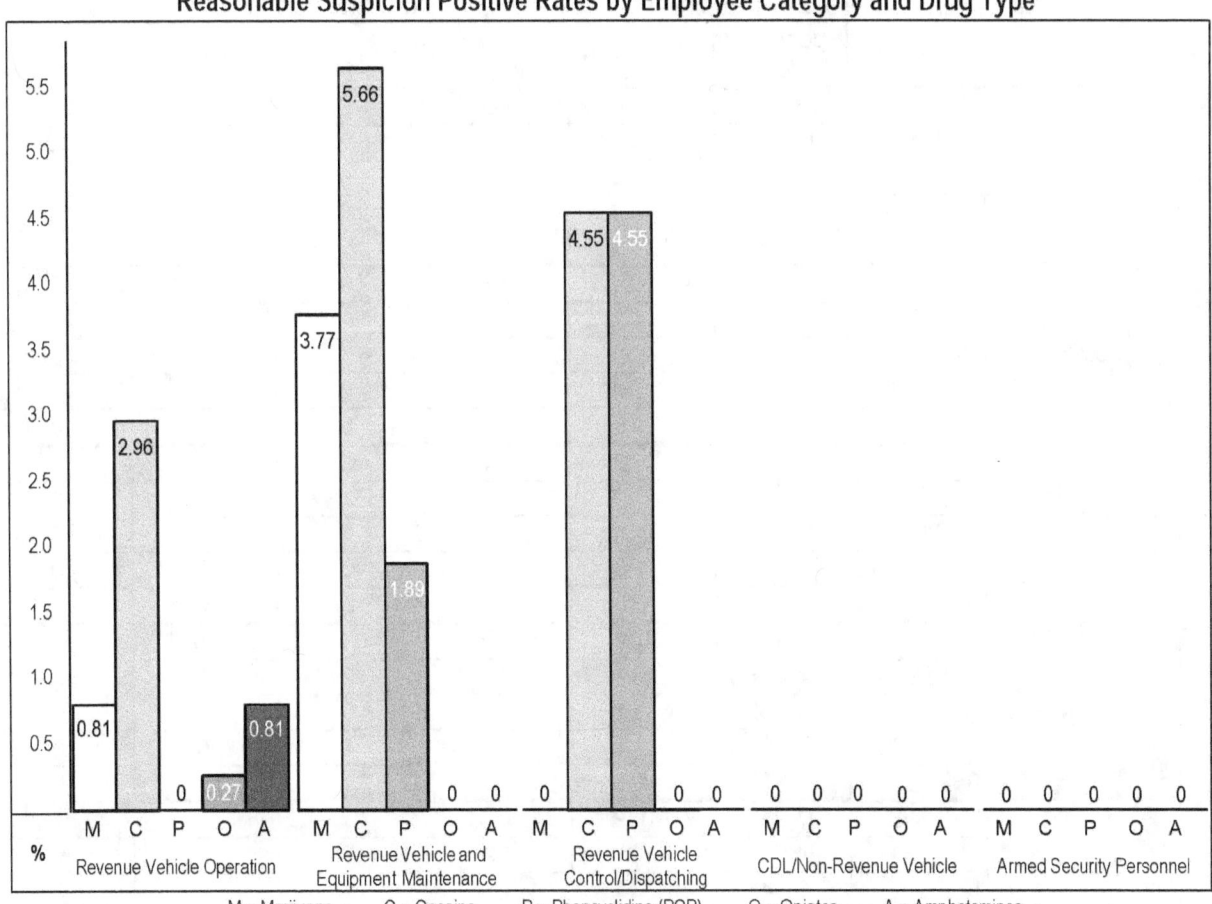

M = Marijuana   C = Cocaine   P = Phencyclidine (PCP)   O = Opiates   A = Amphetamines

Pre-Employment Positive Rates by Employee Category and Drug Type

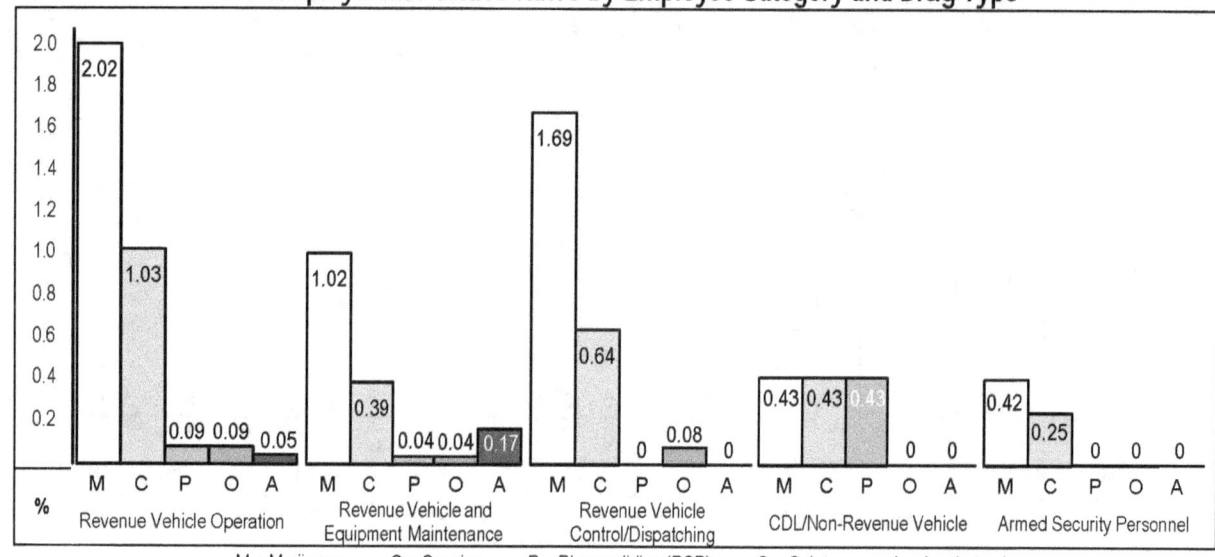

M = Marijuana   C = Cocaine   P = Phencyclidine (PCP)   O = Opiates   A = Amphetamines

Specimens Collected and Positives by Test Type, Employee Category, and Drug Type

		Specimens Collected	Verified Positives				
			Marijuana	Cocaine	PCP	Opiates	Amphetamines
Random	RVO	54,676	270	225	6	15	20
	RV&EM	19,670	85	64	2	7	10
	RVC/D	4,983	13	18	0	1	0
	CDL/N-RV	1,435	8	4	0	0	0
	ASP	1,749	2	2	0	0	0
Post-Accident	RVO	7,617	57	58	0	7	4
	RV&EM	363	5	3	0	0	0
	RVC/D	94	0	0	0	0	0
	CDL/N-RV	33	0	0	0	0	0
	ASP	53	0	0	0	0	0
Reasonable Suspicion	RVO	371	3	11	0	1	3
	RV&EM	53	2	3	1	0	0
	RVC/D	22	0	1	1	0	0
	CDL/N-RV	1	0	0	0	0	0
	ASP	5	0	0	0	0	0
Pre-Employment	RVO	35,152	709	361	31	30	18
	RV&EM	4,818	49	19	2	2	8
	RVC/D	1,242	21	8	0	1	0
	CDL/N-RV	235	1	1	1	0	0
	ASP	1,203	5	3	1	0	0
Total	RVO	97,816	1,039	655	37	53	45
	RV&EM	24,904	141	89	5	9	18
	RVC/D	6,341	34	27	1	2	0
	CDL/N-RV	1,704	9	5	1	0	0
	ASP	3,010	7	5	1	0	0

RVO = Revenue Vehicle Operation   RV&EM = Revenue Vehicle and Equipment Maintenance
RVC/D = Revenue Vehicle Control/Dispatching   CDL/N-RV = CDL/Non-Revenue Vehicle   ASP = Armed Security Personnel

Percentage by Drug Type of Total Drug Detections for Each Test Type by Employee Category

	Revenue Vehicle Operation					Revenue Vehicle and Equipment Maintenance					Revenue Vehicle Control/Dispatching					CDL/Non-Revenue Vehicle					Armed Security Personnel				
	M	C	P	O	A	M	C	P	O	A	M	C	P	O	A	M	C	P	O	A	M	C	P	O	A
Random	50.4	42.0	1.1	2.8	3.7	50.6	38.1	1.2	4.2	5.9	40.6	56.3	0	3.1	0	66.7	33.3	0	0	0	50.0	50.0	0	0	0
Post-Accident	45.2	46.0	0	5.6	3.2	62.5	37.5	0	0	0	0	0	0	0	0	0	0	0	0	0	0	0	0	0	0
Reasonable Suspicion	16.7	61.1	0	5.5	16.7	33.3	50.0	16.7	0	0	0	50.0	50.0	0	0	0	0	0	0	0	0	0	0	0	0
Pre-Employment	61.7	31.4	2.7	2.6	1.6	61.25	23.75	2.5	2.5	10.0	70.0	26.7	0	3.3	0	33.3	33.3	33.3	0	0	55.6	33.3	11.1	0	0
Combined	55.7	37.4	1.1	2.5	3.3	63.3	30.7	3.0	2.0	1.0	52.6	42.1	0	0	5.3	48.4	45.2	3.2	3.2	0	61.5	38.5	0	0	0

M = Marijuana   C = Cocaine   P = Phencyclidine (PCP)   O = Opiates   A = Amphetamines

3.5 Non-Positive Alcohol Violations

Data are presented for alcohol violations other than positive test results:
- Confirmed specimens with breath alcohol levels between 0.02 and 0.039
- Non-test violations:
  - Alcohol use while performing a safety-sensitive function
  - Alcohol use within 4 hours of performing a safety-sensitive function
  - Alcohol use before taking a required post-accident test
  - Other

3.5.1 Confirmed Alcohol Specimens Between 0.02 and 0.039

The following tables present data on confirmed alcohol specimens produced at levels between 0.02 and 0.039 for each test type and for all four test types combined. The data presented are the percentage of such specimens of the total number of screens produced and the statistical basis for those percentages. (For all test types except reasonable suspicion and for all the types combined, the percentages of the entire number of screens and the percentage of the total number with levels lower than 0.04 are the same after rounding because the rates are extremely low. Both rates are included in the "percent of total screens" column for reasonable suspicion tests where the rates differ.)

The table at right presents the total number of violations. The tables on the following pages subdivide those numbers by employer type, by employer size, by employer size and type combined, by employee category, and by FTA region, respectively. The rates by FTA region are presented for all four test types combined and for random tests, but not for the other three test types individually.

Alcohol Confirmations Between 0.02 and 0.039 by Test Type

	Percent of Total Screens	Between 0.02 and 0.039	Total Screens
Random	0.07	19	28,216
Post-Accident	0.03	2	7,759
Reasonable Suspicion	2.35/ 2.54*	11	469
Pre-Employment	0.01	1	9,157
Total	0.07	33	45,601

* The bottom number is the percentage of the total number of screens excluding confirmed positives. Both percentages are the same for the other test types.

Alcohol Confirmations Between 0.02 and 0.039 by Test Type and Employer Type

	Transit			Contractor		
	Percent of Total Screens	Between 0.02 and 0.039	Total Screens	Percent of Total Screens	Between 0.02 and 0.039	Total Screens
Random	0.06	14	23,362	0.10	5	4,854
Post-Accident	0.02	1	6,222	0.07	1	1,537
Reasonable Suspicion	2.78/3.00*	10	360	0.92/1.00*	1	109
Pre-Employment	0.02	1	6,149	0	0	3,008
Total	0.07	26	36,093	0.07	7	9,508

*The bottom number is the percentage of the total number of screens excluding confirmed positives. Both percentages are the same for the other test types.

Alcohol Confirmations Between 0.02 and 0.039 by Test Type and Employer Size

	Large			Small			Rural		
	Percent of Total Screens	Between 0.02 and 0.039	Total Screens	Percent of Total Screens	Between 0.02 and 0.039	Total Screens	Percent of Total Screens	Between 0.02 and 0.039	Total Screens
Random	0.07	19	27,015	0	0	338	0	0	863
Post-Accident	0.03	2	7,501	0	0	100	0	0	158
Reasonable Suspicion	2.17/2.35*	10	461	0	0	3	20.00	1	5
Pre-Employment	0.01	1	8,580	0	0	29	0	0	548
Total	0.07	32	43,557	0	0	470	0.06	1	1,574

*The bottom number is the percentage of the total number of screens excluding confirmed positives. Both percentages are the same for the other reasonable suspicion breakdowns and for the other test types.

Alcohol Confirmations Between 0.02 and 0.039 by Test Type, Employer Size, and Employer Type

	Large						Small						Rural					
	Transit			Contractor			Transit			Contractor			Transit			Contractor		
	%TS	.02-.039	TS	%TS	.02-.039	TS	%TS	.02-.039	TS	%TS	.02-.039	TS	%TS	.02-.039	TS	%TS	.02-.039	TS
Random	0.06	14	22,396	0.11	5	4,619	0	0	290	0	0	48	0	0	676	0	0	187
Post-Accident	0.02	1	6,016	0.07	1	1,485	0	0	85	0	0	15	0	0	121	0	0	37
Reasonable Suspicion	2.54/2.74*	9	355	0.94/1.03*	1	106	0	0	2	0	0	1	33.33	1	3		0	0
Pre-Employment	0.02	1	5,873	0	0	2,707	0	0	22	0	0	7	0	0	254	0	0	294
Total	0.07	25	34,640	0.08	7	8,917	0	0	399	0	0	71	0.09	1	1,054		0	520

TS = total screens   *The bottom number is the percentage of the total number of screens excluding confirmed positives. Both percentages are the same for the other reasonable suspicion breakdowns and for the other test types.

Alcohol Confirmations Between 0.02 and 0.039 by Test Type and Employee Category

	Revenue Vehicle Operation			Revenue Vehicle and Equipment Maintenance			Revenue Vehicle Control/Dispatching			CDL/Non-Revenue Vehicle			Armed Security Personnel		
	Percent of Total Screens	0.02 to 0.039	Total Screens	Percent of Total Screens	0.02 to 0.039	Total Screens	Percent of Total Screens	0.02 to 0.039	Total Screens	Percent of Total Screens	0.02 to 0.039	Total Screens	Percent of Total Screens	0.02 to 0.039	Total Screens
Random	0.04	8	18,485	0.10	7	6,812	0.20	3	1,506	0.14	1	696	0	0	717
Post-Accident	0.03	2	7,243	0	0	342	0	0	91	0	0	32	0	0	51
Reasonable Suspicion	2.58/2.80*	10	388	0	0	54	0	0	22	100	1	1	0	0	4
Pre-Employment	0.01	1	7,152	0	0	1,278	0	0	270	0	0	63	0	0	394
Total	0.06	21	33,268	0.08	7	8,486	0.16	3	1,889	0.25	2	792	0	0	1,166

*The bottom number is the percentage of the total number of screens excluding confirmed positives. Both percentages are the same for the other reasonable suspicion breakdowns and for the other test types.

Random Alcohol Confirmations Between 0.02 and 0.039 by FTA Region			
Region	Percent of Total Screens	Between 0.02 and 0.039	Total Screens
1	0	0	621
2	0.04	3	7,501
3	0.10	5	5,256
4	0.03	1	3,950
5	0.07	2	2,734
6	0.10	3	3,060
7	0.37	1	268
8	0	0	593
9	0	0	2,169
10	0.19	4	2,064

Total Alcohol Confirmations Between 0.02 and 0.039 for Four Test Types Combined by FTA Region			
Region	Percent of Total Screens	Between 0.02 and 0.039	Total Screens
1	0	0	877
2	0.04	4	11,235
3	0.05	5	9,216
4	0.03	2	6,538
5	0.11	5	4,690
6	0.11	5	4,412
7	0.83	4	483
8	0	0	875
9	0.06	3	4,759
10	0.20	5	2,516

3.5.2 Non-Test Alcohol Violations

Because non-test violations cannot be expressed as a rate, the number of instances reported have been normalized for all employers by each size category. Data are provided for each of three specific non-test violations and for non-test violations that were not classified. The first table presents the total number of violations. The other tables subdivide those numbers by employer type and employer size, respectively. The table of violations by size also subdivides the large employer data by employer type. Non-test violations were not reported by employee category.

Non-Test Alcohol Violations	Normalized	Reported
Alcohol use while performing a safety-sensitive function	10	6
Alcohol use within 4 hours of performing a safety-sensitive function	6	4
Alcohol use before taking a required post-accident test	0	0
Unclassified non-test violations	5	3
Total	16	10

Non-Test Alcohol Violations by Employer Type	Normalized		Reported	
	Transit	Contractor	Transit	Contractor
Alcohol use while performing a safety-sensitive function	8	2	5	1
Alcohol use within 4 hours of performing a safety-sensitive function	5	1	3	1
Unclassified non-test violations	2	3	1	2
Total	13	6	8	4

Non-Test Alcohol Violations by Employer Size	Normalized			Small	Rural	Reported			Small	Rural
	Large Total	T	C			Large Total	T	C		
Alcohol use while performing a safety-sensitive function	10	8	2	0	0	6	5	1	0	0
Alcohol use within 4 hours of performing a safety-sensitive function	6	5	1	0	0	4	3	1	0	0
Unclassified non-test violations	5	2	3	0	0	3	1	2	0	0
Total	21	15	6	0	0	13	9	4	0	0

T = transit   C = contractor

4. Return to Duty Data

This chapter presents data on persons who have been returned to FTA safety-sensitive duty after testing positive for drugs or alcohol or refusing to submit to a required test and who have subsequently completed a rehabilitation program designed by a substance abuse professional (SAP). Section 4.1 presents statistics on the number of persons returned to duty in calendar year 2002. Section 4.2 summarizes data for return to duty tests performed in 2002. Section 4.3 summarizes data for follow-up tests performed in 2002. The results are sorted and presented by various criteria: employer type, employer size, employee category, FTA region, and drug type.

As mentioned in Chapter 1, only a portion of the recipients and subrecipients were requested to report their test data in 2002. Those employers were randomly selected from three stratified sample populations, based on employer size—535 large employers, 36 small employers, and 237 rural employers.[8] To make the sample data meaningful, the results are expressed as rates where possible, i.e., in Sections 4.2 and 4.3. In Section 4.1, where the data cannot be expressed as a rate, the number of instances reported have been normalized for the total number of employees by each size category to represent the total number of employers. The number of instances reported is also presented to provide basis for the rates or normalization.

4.1 Employees Returned to Duty in 2002

Data are presented for the number of employees who were returned to duty following a drug violation and following an alcohol violation. However, one person may test positive for both drugs and alcohol, and most employers test the returned employees for both drugs and alcohol. Thus, the numbers for drugs and alcohol cannot be added to obtain the total number of persons returned to duty. No statistics were reported for the total number returned to duty.

Employees Returned to Duty

	Drugs	Alcohol
Normalized	677	98
Reported	358	52

The table at left presents the number of employees returned to duty. These data are subdivided by employer type and by employer size in the tables below. The data by employer size are further subdivided by employer type on the next page. Employees returned to duty were not reported by employee category.

Employees Returned to Duty by Employer Type

	Drugs		Alcohol	
	Transit	Contractor	Transit	Contractor
Normalized	569	108	82	16
Reported	326	32	45	7

Employees Returned to Duty by Employer Size

	Drugs			Alcohol		
	Large	Small	Rural	Large	Small	Rural
Normalized	560	93	24	80	0	18
Reported	345	9	4	49	0	3

---

[8] The population that surrounds the transit organization determines the employer size category. Large is 200,000 or more, small is 50,000 to 200,000, and rural is less than 50,000.

Employees Returned to Duty by Employer Size and Employer Type

	Drugs						Alcohol					
	Large		Small		Rural		Large		Small		Rural	
	Transit	Contractor	Transit	Contractor	Transit	Contractor	Transit	Contractor	Transit	Contractor	Transit	Contractor
Normalized	520	40	31	62	18	6	70	10	0	0	12	6
Reported	320	25	3	6	3	1	43	6	0	0	2	1

4.2 Return to Duty Test Data

The positive rates for return to duty drug tests and alcohol tests[9] are shown in the graph at left. The statistical basis for those rates is provided in the table. The rates are subdivided by employer type and size, by employee category, by FTA region, and by type of drug later in this section.

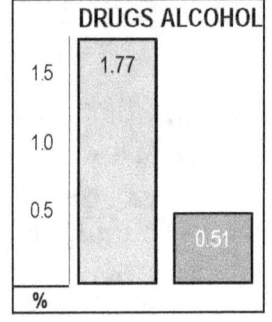

Return to Duty Positive Rates

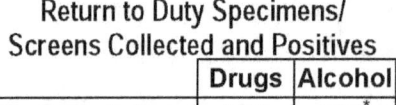

Return to Duty Specimens/ Screens Collected and Positives

	Drugs	Alcohol
Specimens Collected	623	396[*]
Verified Positives	11	2[**]

*Total screens collected **Confirmed Positives

4.2.1 Return to Duty Test Data by Employer Type and Size

The following three graphs present the return to duty drug test and alcohol test rates by employer type, employer size, and employer size and type, respectively. Two of the rates in two of the graphs are presented on a separate scale because their sample sizes are too small to be representative of their populations. The graph (at right) showing employer size rates subdivided by employer type shows alcohol rates only for large transit employers because no confirmed alcohol positives were reported by small or rural employers or by contractors. The three tables that follow provide the statistical basis for the positive rates.

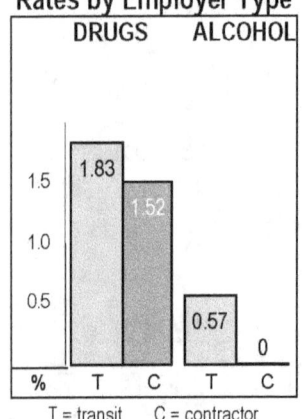

Return to Duty Positive Rates by Employer Type

T = transit   C = contractor

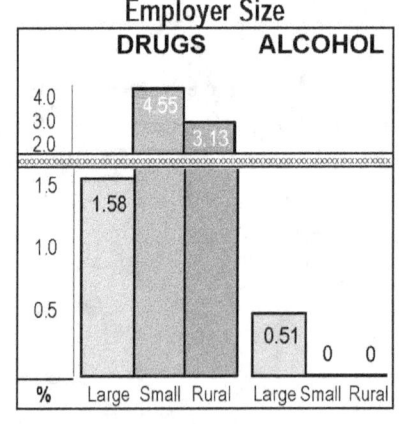

Return to Duty Positive Rates by Employer Size

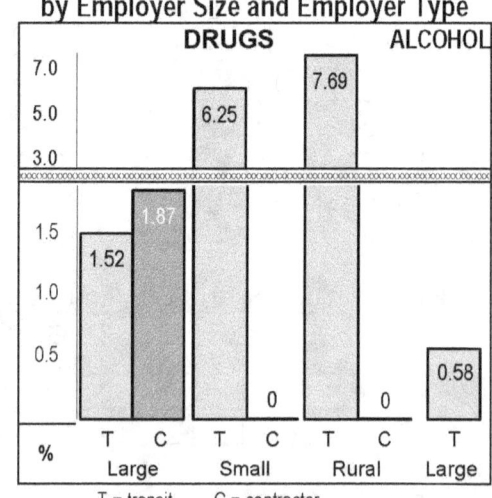

Return to Duty Positive Rates by Employer Size and Employer Type

T = transit   C = contractor

[9]A positive alcohol test is a screen with a confirmed breath alcohol level of at least 0.04.

	Drugs		Alcohol	
	Transit	Contractor	Transit	Contractor
Specimens Collected	491	132	351*	45*
Verified Positives	9	2	2**	0**

Return to Duty Specimens/Screens Collected and Positives by Employer Type

*Total screens collected   **Confirmed Positives

	Drugs			Alcohol		
	Large	Small	Rural	Large	Small	Rural
Specimens Collected	569	22	32	390*	4*	2*
Verified Positives	9	1	1	2**	0**	0**

Return to Duty Specimens/Screens Collected and Positives by Employer Size

*Total screens collected   **Confirmed Positives

Return to Duty Specimens/Screens Collected and Positives by Employer Size and Employer Type

	Drugs						Alcohol					
	Large		Small		Rural		Large		Small		Rural	
	Transit	Contractor	Transit	Contractor	Transit	Contractor	Transit	Contractor	Transit	Contractor	Transit	Contractor
Specimens Collected	462	107	16	6	13	19	347*	43*	3*	1*	1*	1*
Verified Positives	7	2	1	0	1	0	2**	0**	0**	0**	0**	0**

*Total screens collected   **Confirmed Positives

4.2.2 Return to Duty Test Data by Employee Category

The following graph shows the verified positive rates for return to duty drug tests and alcohol tests by employee category. The table next to it provides the statistical basis for the positive rates. These data are further subdivided by employer type and by employer size on the next page.

Return to Duty Positive Rates by Employee Category

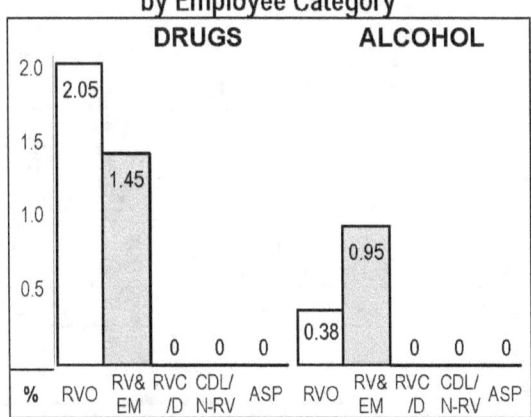

RVO = Revenue Vehicle Operation
RV&EM = Revenue Vehicle and Equipment Maintenance
RVC/D = Revenue Vehicle Control/Dispatching
CDL/N-RV = CDL/Non-Revenue Vehicle
ASP = Armed Security Personnel

Return to Duty Specimens/Screens Collected and Positives by Employee Category

	Drugs	
	Specimens Collected	Verified Positives
Revenue Vehicle Operation	438	9
Revenue Vehicle & Equipment Maintenance	138	2
Revenue Vehicle Control/Dispatching	30	0
CDL/Non-Revenue Vehicle	14	0
Armed Security Personnel	3	0

	Alcohol	
	Screens	Confirmed Positives
Revenue Vehicle Operation	263	1
Revenue Vehicle & Equipment Maintenance	105	1
Revenue Vehicle Control/Dispatching	19	0
CDL/Non-Revenue Vehicle	8	0
Armed Security Personnel	1	0

Note: The graphs subdivided by employer type and employer size do not contain columns for employee categories that show a positive rate of "0" in the preceding employee category graph.

Return to Duty Positive Rates by Employee Category and Employer Type

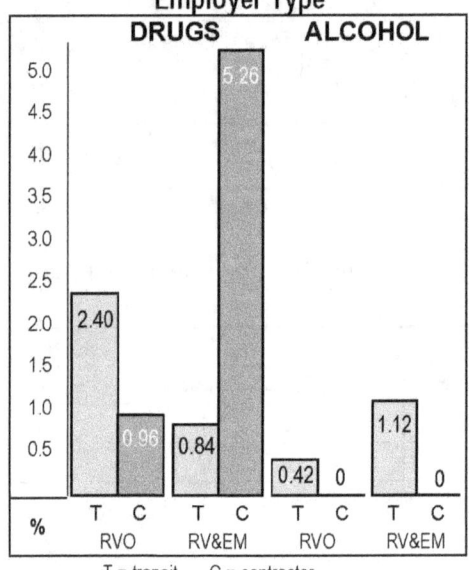

T = transit   C = contractor
RVO = Revenue Vehicle Operation
RV&EM = Revenue Vehicle and Equipment Maintenance

Return to Duty Specimens/Screens Collected and Positives by Employee Category and Employer Type

	Drugs			
	Transit		Contractor	
	SC	VP	SC	VP
Revenue Vehicle Operation	334	8	104	1
Revenue Vehicle & Equipment Maintenance	119	1	19	1
Revenue Vehicle Control/Dispatching	25	0	5	0
CDL/Non-Revenue Vehicle	10	0	4	0
Armed Security Personnel	3	0	0	0

	Alcohol			
	Transit		Contractor	
	S	CP	S	CP
Revenue Vehicle Operation	238	1	25	0
Revenue Vehicle & Equipment Maintenance	89	1	16	0
Revenue Vehicle Control/Dispatching	16	0	3	0
CDL/Non-Revenue Vehicle	7	0	1	0
Armed Security Personnel	1	0	0	0

SC = specimens collected   VP = verified positives
S = screens   CP = confirmed positives

Two of the rates in the next graph are presented on a separate scale because their sample sizes are too small to be representative of their populations. Additionally, that graph contains alcohol rate columns for only large employers because no positive return to duty alcohol tests were reported by small or rural employers in 2002.

Return to Duty Positive Rates by Employee Category and Employer Size

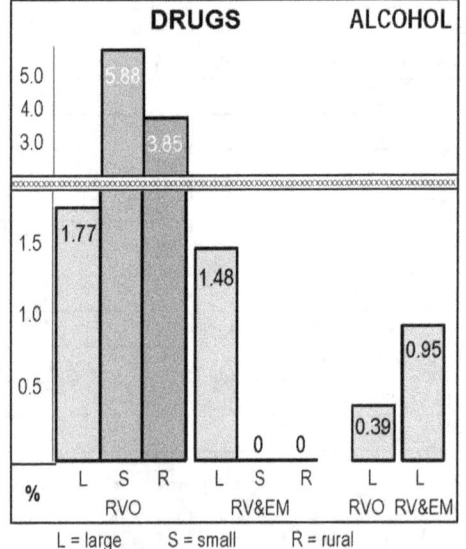

L = large   S = small   R = rural
RVO = Revenue Vehicle Operation
RV&EM = Revenue Vehicle and Equipment Maintenance

Return to Duty Specimens/Screens Collected and Positives by Employee Category and Employer Size

	Drugs					
	Large		Small		Rural	
	SC	VP	SC	VP	SC	VP
Revenue Vehicle Operation	395	7	17	1	26	1
Revenue Vehicle & Equipment Maintenance	135	2	1	0	2	0
Revenue Vehicle Control/Dispatching	24	0	3	0	3	0
CDL/Non-Revenue Vehicle	13	0	0	0	1	0
Armed Security Personnel	2	0	1	0	0	0

	Alcohol					
	Large		Small		Rural	
	S	CP	S	CP	S	CP
Revenue Vehicle Operation	258	1	3	0	2	0
Revenue Vehicle & Equipment Maintenance	105	1	0	0	0	0
Revenue Vehicle Control/Dispatching	18	0	1	0	0	0
CDL/Non-Revenue Vehicle	8	0	0	0	0	0
Armed Security Personnel	1	0	0	0	0	0

SC = specimens collected   VP = verified positives
S = screens   CP = confirmed positives

4.2.3 Return to Duty Test Data by FTA Region

The following map shows the verified positive rates for return to duty drug tests for each of FTA's ten regions. The shading variations enable quick comparison. The exact rates are also included. The statistical basis for those rates is provided in the accompanying table. Because only two return to duty alcohol positives were reported, the alcohol rates for each region appear in a table (below the map), along with the statistical basis for those rates.

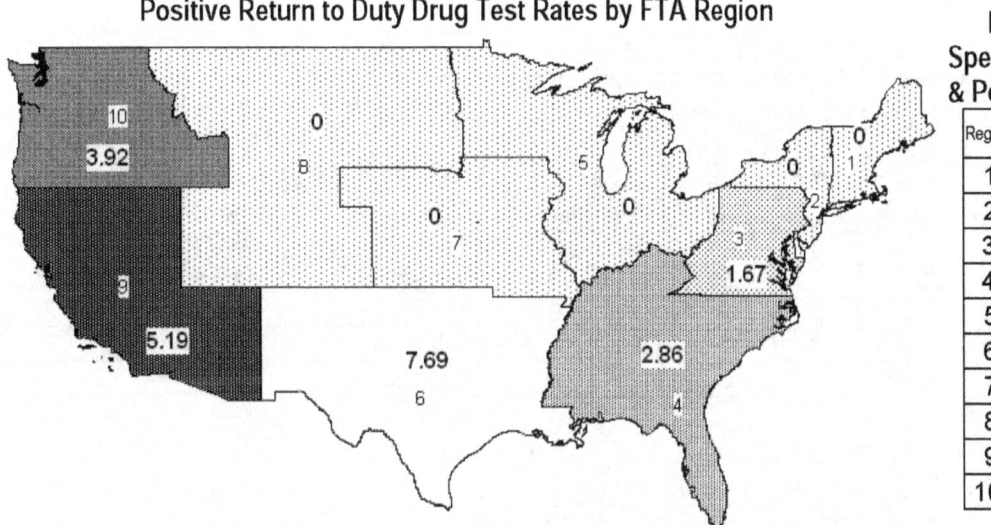

Positive Return to Duty Drug Test Rates by FTA Region

Return to Duty Specimens Collected & Positives by Region

Region	Specimens Collected	Verified Positives
1	16	0
2	140	0
3	120	2
4	35	1
5	129	0
6	26	2
7	13	0
8	16	0
9	77	4
10	51	2

Return to Duty Alcohol Data by FTA Region

Region	1	2	3	4	5	6	7	8	9	10
Positive Rate	0	0	1.90	0	0	0	0	0	0	0
Screens	12	78	105	25	65	19	9	15	53	15
Confirmed Positives	0	0	2	0	0	0	0	0	0	0

4.2.4 Return to Duty Test Data by Type of Drug

The next two tables show return to duty test data for each type of drug tested for. The number of drug test specimens collected and the number and percent of those that were verified positive are shown at left. The percentage of total positives by drug type are shown at right. These data are subdivided by employer type, by employer size, and by employee category on the next page.

Return to Duty Specimens Collected, Positives, and Rates by Drug Type

623 specimens collected		
	Positives	Percent
Marijuana	6	0.96
Cocaine	4	0.64
PCP	0	0
Opiates	0	0
Amphetamines	1	0.16

Percentage by Drug Type for Return to Duty Positives

Marijuana	54.5
Cocaine	36.4
PCP	0
Opiates	0
Amphetamines	9.1

Return to Duty Specimens Collected, Positives, and Rates by Drug Type and Employer Type

	Transit		Contractor	
	491 collected		132 collected	
	Positives	Percent	Positives	Percent
Marijuana	4	0.81	2	1.52
Cocaine	4	0.81	0	0
PCP	0	0	0	0
Opiates	0	0	0	0
Amphetamines	1	0.20	0	0

Percentage by Drug Type for Return to Duty Positives by Employer Type

	Transit	Contractor
Marijuana	44.45	100
Cocaine	44.45	0
PCP	0	0
Opiates	0	0
Amphetamines	11.1	0

Return to Duty Specimens Collected, Positives, and Rates by Drug Type and Employer Size

	Large		Small		Rural	
	569 collected		22 collected		32 collected	
	Positives	Percent	Positives	Percent	Positives	Percent
Marijuana	5	0.88	0	0	1	3.13
Cocaine	3	0.53	1	4.55	0	0
PCP	0	0	0	0	0	0
Opiates	0	0	0	0	0	0
Amphetamines	1	0.18	0	0	0	0

Percentage by Drug Type for Return to Duty Positives by Employer Size

	Large	Small	Rural
Marijuana	55.6	0	100
Cocaine	33.3	100	0
PCP	11.1	0	0
Opiates	0	0	0
Amphetamines	0	0	0

Return to Duty Specimens Collected, Positives, and Rates by Drug Type and Employee Category

	RVO		RV&EM		RVC/D		CDL/N-RV		ASP	
	438 collected		138 collected		30 collected		14 collected		3 collected	
	Positives	Percent	Positives	Percent	Positives	Percent	Positives	Percent	Positives	Percent
Marijuana	5	1.14	1	0.72	0	0	0	0	0	0
Cocaine	3	0.68	1	0.72	0	0	0	0	0	0
PCP	0	0	0	0	0	0	0	0	0	0
Opiates	0	0	0	0	0	0	0	0	0	0
Amphetamines	1	0.23	0	0	0	0	0	0	0	0

Percentage by Drug Type for Return to Duty Positives by Employee Category

	RVO	RV&EM	RVC/D	CDL/N-RV	ASP
M	55.6		0	0	0
C	33.3	0	0	0	0
P	0	0	0	0	0
O	0	0	0	0	0
A	11.1	0	0	0	0

RVO = Revenue Vehicle Operation RV&EM = Revenue Vehicle and Equipment Maintenance
RVC/D = Revenue Vehicle Control/Dispatching CDL/N-RV = CDL/Non-Revenue Vehicle ASP = Armed Security Personnel
M = Marijuana C = Cocaine P = Phencyclidine (PCP) O = Opiates A = Amphetamines

4.3 Follow-Up Test Data

Follow-Up Positive Rates

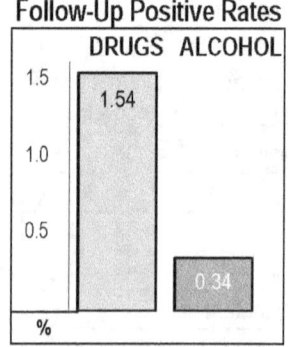

The positive rates for follow-up drug tests and alcohol tests are shown in the graph at left. The statistical basis for those rates is provided in the table below. These data are subdivided by employer type and size, by employee category, by FTA region, and by type of drug later in this section.

Follow-Up Specimens/Screens Collected and Positives

	Drugs	Alcohol
Specimens Collected	5,502	4,389*
Verified Positives	85	15**

*Total screens collected **Confirmed Positives

4.3.1 Follow-Up Test Data by Employer Type and Size

The following three graphs present the follow-up test rates by employer type, by employer size, and by employer size and type, respectively. Rates in two of the graphs are presented on a separate scale because their sample sizes are too small to be representative of their populations. The graph (at right) showing employer size rates subdivided by employer type shows alcohol rates only for large employers because no confirmed alcohol positives were reported by small or rural employers. The three tables that follow provide the statistical basis for the positive rates.

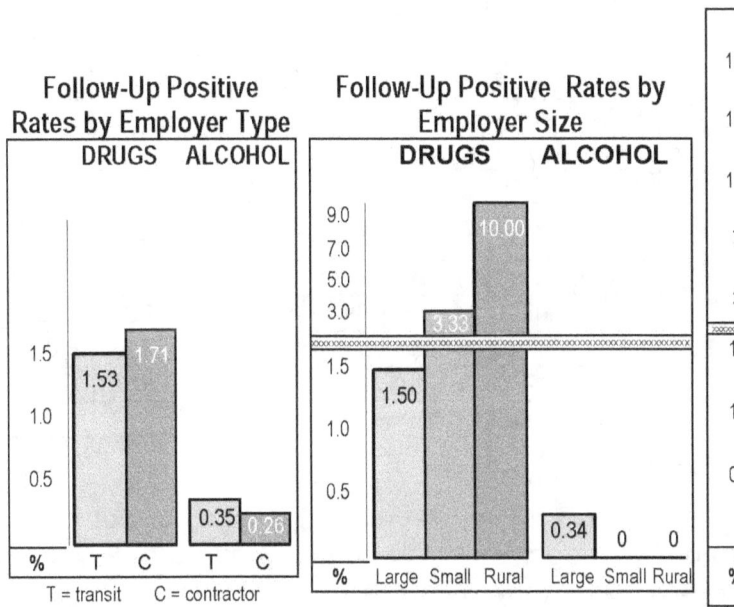

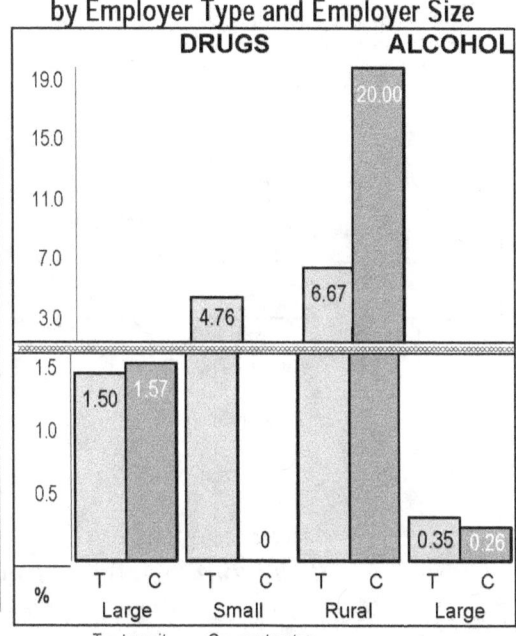

Follow-Up Specimens/Screens Collected and Positives by Employer Type

	Drugs		Alcohol	
	Transit	Contractor	Transit	Contractor
Specimens Collected	4,977	525	3,997[*]	392[*]
Verified Positives	76	9	14[**]	1[**]

*Total screens collected   **Confirmed Positives

Follow-Up Specimens/Screens Collected and Positives by Employer Size

	Drugs			Alcohol		
	Large	Small	Rural	Large	Small	Rural
Specimens Collected	5,452	30	20	4,368[*]	9[*]	12[*]
Verified Positives	82	1	2	15[**]	0[**]	0[**]

*Total screens collected   **Confirmed Positives

Follow-Up Specimens/Screens Collected and Positives by Employer Size and Employer Type

	Drugs						Alcohol					
	Large		Small		Rural		Large		Small		Rural	
	Transit	Contractor	Transit	Contractor	Transit	Contractor	Transit	Contractor	Transit	Contractor	Transit	Contractor
Specimens Collected	4,941	511	21	9	15	5	3,989[*]	379[*]	1[*]	8[*]	7[*]	5[*]
Verified Positives	74	8	1	0	1	1	14[**]	1[**]	0[**]	0[**]	0[**]	0[**]

*Total screens collected   **Confirmed Positives

4.3.2 Follow-Up Test Data by Employee Category

The following graph shows the positive rates for follow-up drug tests and alcohol tests by employee category. The accompanying table provides the statistical basis for the positive rates. These data are further subdivided by employer type and employer size in the subsequent graphs and tables.

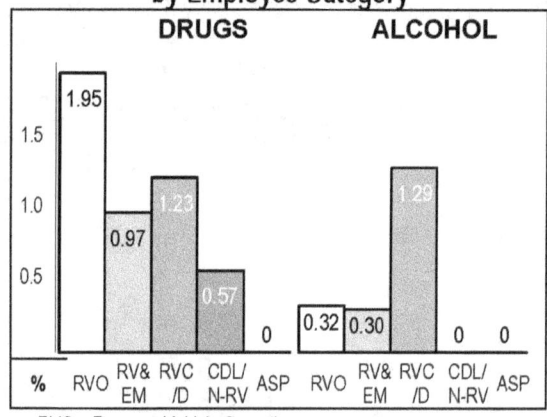

Follow-Up Positive Rates by Employee Category

RVO = Revenue Vehicle Operation
RV&EM = Revenue Vehicle and Equipment Maintenance
RVC/D = Revenue Vehicle Control/Dispatching
CDL/N-RV = CDL/Non-Revenue Vehicle

Follow-Up Specimens/Screens Collected and Positives by Employee Category

	Drugs	
	Specimens Collected	Verified Positives
Revenue Vehicle Operation	3,223	63
Revenue Vehicle & Equipment Maintenance	1,849	18
Revenue Vehicle Control/Dispatching	244	3
CDL/Non-Revenue Vehicle	175	1
Armed Security Personnel	11	0

	Alcohol	
	Screens	Confirmed Positives
Revenue Vehicle Operation	2,477	8
Revenue Vehicle & Equipment Maintenance	1,651	5
Revenue Vehicle Control/Dispatching	155	2
CDL/Non-Revenue Vehicle	102	0
Armed Security Personnel	4	0

Note: The graphs subdivided by employer type and employer size do not contain columns for employee categories that show a positive rate of "0" in the preceding employee category graph.

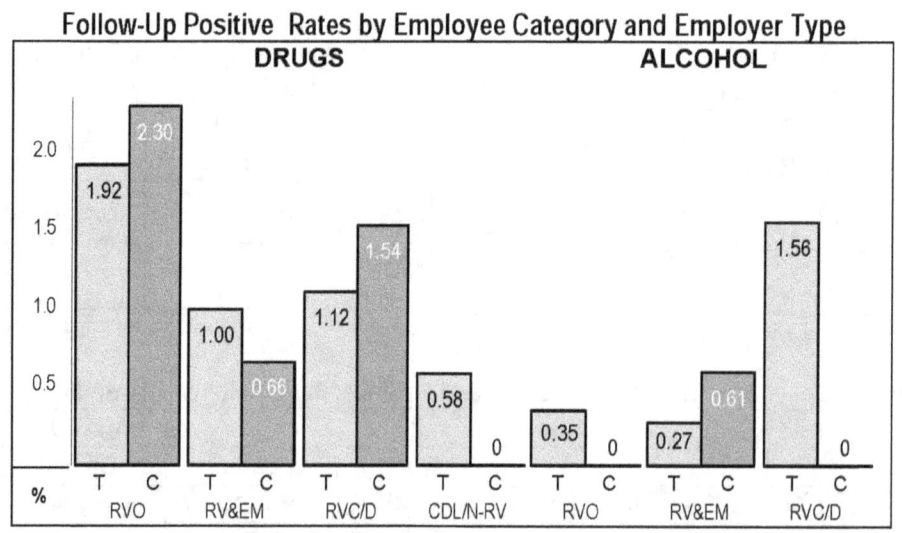

Follow-Up Positive Rates by Employee Category and Employer Type

T = transit   C = contractor

RVO = Revenue Vehicle Operation
RVC/D = Revenue Vehicle Control/Dispatching

RV&EM = Revenue Vehicle and Equipment Maintenance
CDL/N-RV = CDL/Non-Revenue Vehicle

Follow-Up Specimens/Screens Collected and Positives by Employee Category and Employer Type

	Drugs				Alcohol			
	Transit		Contractor		Transit		Contractor	
	Specimens Collected	Verified Positives	Specimens Collected	Verified Positives	Screens	Confirmed Positives	Screens	Confirmed Positives
Revenue Vehicle Operation	2,918	56	305	7	2,278	8	199	0
Revenue Vehicle and Equipment Maintenance	1,698	17	151	1	1,486	4	165	1
Revenue Vehicle Control/Dispatching	179	2	65	1	128	2	27	0
CDL/Non-Revenue Vehicle	171	1	4	0	101	0	1	0
Armed Security Personnel	11	0	0	0	4	0	0	0

Two of the rates in the next graph are presented on a separate scale because their sample sizes are too small to be representative of their populations. Additionally, that graph contains alcohol rate columns for only large employers because no positive follow-up alcohol tests were reported by small or rural employers.

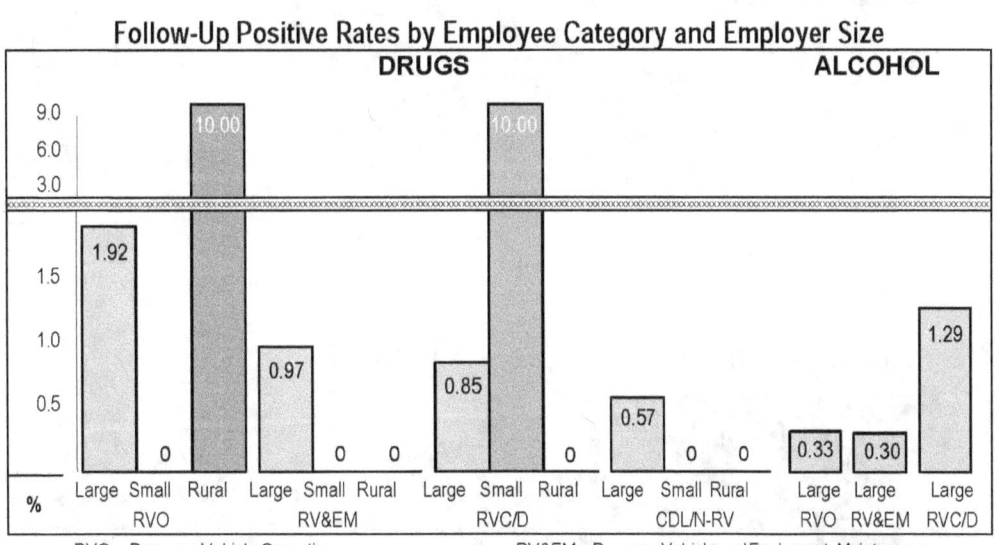

Follow-Up Positive Rates by Employee Category and Employer Size

RVO = Revenue Vehicle Operation
RVC/D = Revenue Vehicle Control/Dispatching
RV&EM = Revenue Vehicle and Equipment Maintenance
CDL/N-RV = CDL/Non-Revenue Vehicle

Follow-Up Specimens/Screens Collected and Positives by Employee Category and Employer Size

	Drugs						Alcohol					
	Large		Small		Rural		Large		Small		Rural	
	Specimens Collected	Verified Positives	Specimens Collected	Verified Positives	Specimens Collected	Verified Positives	Screens	Confirmed Positives	Screens	Confirmed Positives	Screens	Confirmed Positives
Revenue Vehicle Operation	3,183	61	20	0	20	2	2,456	8	9	0	12	0
Revenue Vehicle and Equipment Maintenance	1,849	18	0	0	0	0	1,651	5	0	0	0	0
Revenue Vehicle Control/Dispatching	234	2	10	1	0	0	155	2	0	0	0	0
CDL/Non-Revenue Vehicle	175	1	0	0	0	0	102	0	0	0	0	0
Armed Security Personnel	11	0	0	0	0	0	4	0	0	0	0	0

4.3.3 Follow-Up Test Data by FTA Region

The following two maps show the positive rates for follow-up drug tests and alcohol tests for each of FTA's ten regions. The shading variations enable quick comparison. The exact rates are also included. The statistical basis for those rates is provided in the accompanying tables.

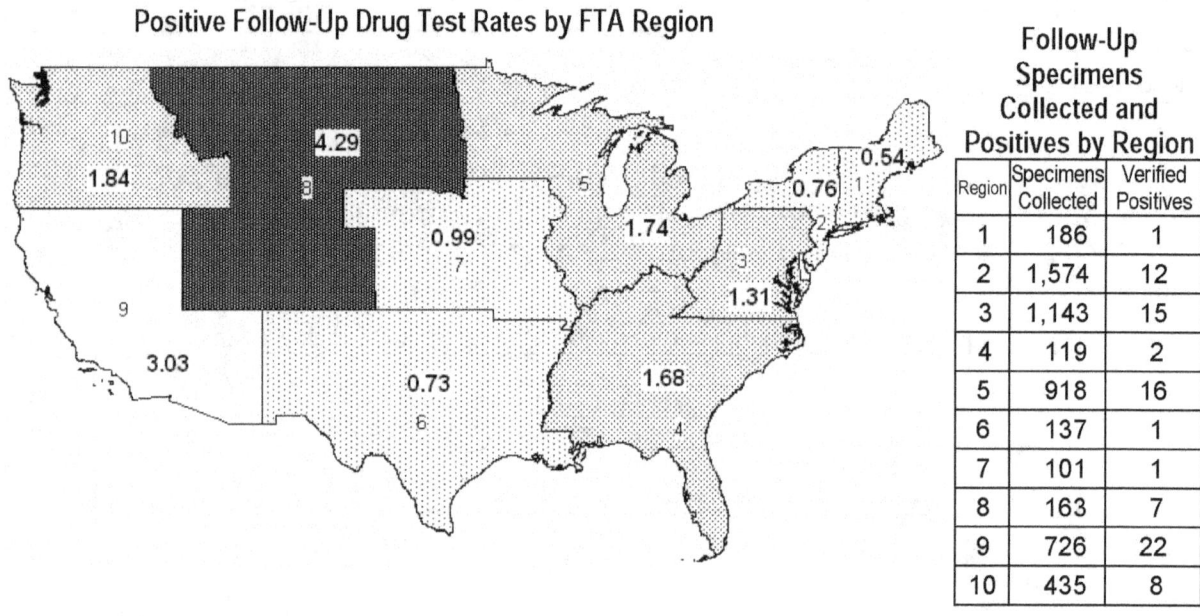

Positive Follow-Up Drug Test Rates by FTA Region

Follow-Up Specimens Collected and Positives by Region

Region	Specimens Collected	Verified Positives
1	186	1
2	1,574	12
3	1,143	15
4	119	2
5	918	16
6	137	1
7	101	1
8	163	7
9	726	22
10	435	8

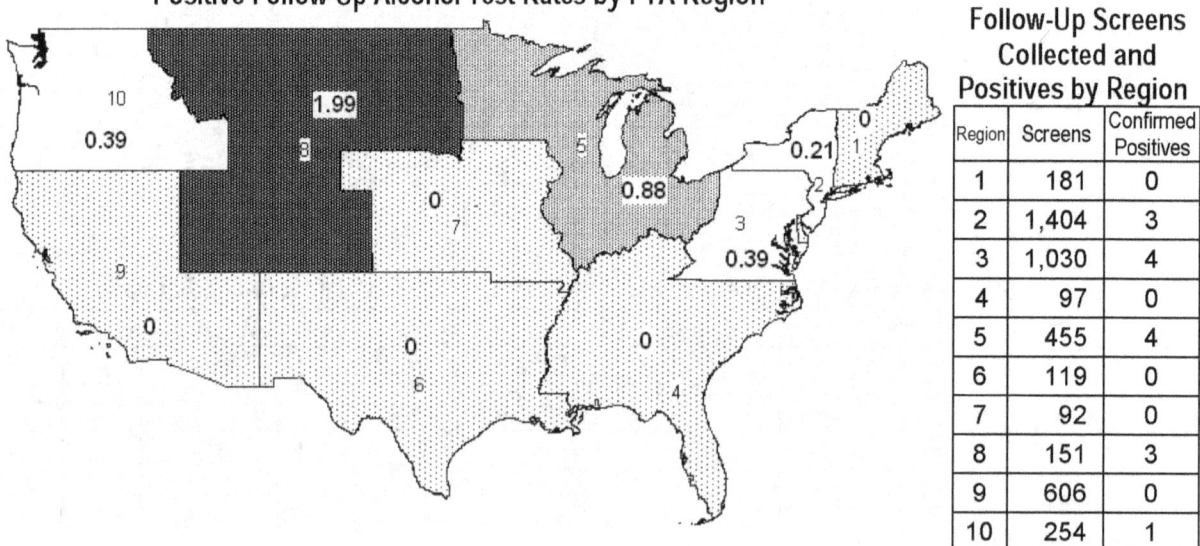

Positive Follow-Up Alcohol Test Rates by FTA Region

Follow-Up Screens Collected and Positives by Region

Region	Screens	Confirmed Positives
1	181	0
2	1,404	3
3	1,030	4
4	97	0
5	455	4
6	119	0
7	92	0
8	151	3
9	606	0
10	254	1

4.3.4 Follow-Up Test Data by Type of Drug

The next two tables show follow-up test data for each type of drug tested for. The number of drug test specimens collected and the number and percent of those that were verified positive are shown at left, and the percentage of total positives by drug type are shown at right. These data are subdivided by employer type, by employer size, and by employee category in the tables that follow.

Follow-Up Specimens Collected, Positives, and Rates by Drug Type

5,502 specimens collected		
	Positives	Percent
Marijuana	39	0.71
Cocaine	41	0.75
PCP	0	0
Opiates	1	0.02
Amphetamines	4	0.07

Percentage by Drug Type for Follow-Up Positives

Marijuana	45.9
Cocaine	48.2
PCP	0
Opiates	1.2
Amphetamines	4.7

Follow-Up Specimens Collected, Positives, and Rates by Drug Type and Employer Type

	Transit		Contractor	
	4,977 collected		525 collected	
	Positives	Percent	Positives	Percent
Marijuana	37	0.74	2	0.38
Cocaine	35	0.70	6	1.14
PCP	0	0	0	0
Opiates	1	0.02	0	0
Amphetamines	3	0.06	1	0.19

Percentage by Drug Type for Follow-Up Positives by Employer Type

	Transit	Contractor
Marijuana	48.7	22.2
Cocaine	46.1	66.7
PCP	0	0
Opiates	1.3	0
Amphetamines	3.9	11.1

Follow-Up Specimens Collected, Positives, and Rates by Drug Type and Employer Size

	Large		Small		Rural	
	5,452 collected		30 collected		20 collected	
	Positives	Percent	Positives	Percent	Positives	Percent
Marijuana	38	0.70	1	3.33	0	0
Cocaine	40	0.73	0	0	1	5.00
PCP	0	0	0	0	0	0
Opiates	1	0.02	0	0	0	0
Amphetamines	3	0.06	0	0	1	5.00

Percentage by Drug Type for Follow-Up Positives by Employer Size

	Large	Small	Rural
Marijuana	46.3	100	0
Cocaine	48.8	0	50.0
PCP	0	0	0
Opiates	1.2	0	0
Amphetamines	3.7	0	50.0

Follow-Up Specimens Collected, Positives, and Rates by Drug Type and Employee Category

	RVO		RV&EM		RVC/D		CDL/N-RV		ASP	
	3223 collected		1849 collected		244 collected		175 collected		11 collected	
	Positives	Percent	Positives	Percent	Positives	Percent	Positives	Percent	Positives	Percent
Marijuana	29	0.90	7	0.38	3	1.23	0	0	0	0
Cocaine	30	0.93	10	0.54	0	0	1	0.57	0	0
PCP	0	0	0	0	0	0	0	0	0	0
Opiates	1	0.03	0	0	0	0	0	0	0	0
Amphetamines	3	0.09	1	0.05	0	0	0	0	0	0

Percentage by Drug Type for Follow-Up Positives by Employee Category

	RVO	RV&EM	RVC/D	CDL/N-RV	ASP
M	46.0	38.9	100	0	0
C	47.6	55.5	0	100	0
P	0	0	0	0	0
O	1.6	0	0	0	0
A	4.8	5.6	0	0	0

RVO = Revenue Vehicle Operation   RV&EM = Revenue Vehicle and Equipment Maintenance
RVC/D = Revenue Vehicle Control/Dispatching   CDL/N-RV = CDL/Non-Revenue Vehicle   ASP = Armed Security Personnel
M = Marijuana   C = Cocaine   P = Phencyclidine (PCP)   O = Opiates   A = Amphetamines

5. Trend Analysis

Because the data reporting requirement changed in 2001, the only rates that can be reliably compared for each year of reporting (from 1996 to 2002) are random violation rates. As mentioned in Chapter 3, the results actually reported in 2001 and 2002 do not accurately reflect total FTA testing due to the high proportion of results reported by large employers. The results from random testing were weighted to obtain "official" random violation rates that reasonably estimate the rate for all persons tested, enabling reliable comparison with the years before 2001 when all employers were required to report. Weighted rates are not available for any test types other than random or any subsets of the random testing.

Also included in this chapter are comparisons of the following rates from results actually reported in 2001 and 2002:

- Random test violation rates subdivided by employer type
- Positive rates for four test types combined: random, post-accident, reasonable suspicion, and pre-employment.

In this report, the violation rate[10] refers to the number of positives and refusals combined per person selected to take a random test:

Drug violation rate = (verified positives + refusals) ÷ (specimens collected + refusals)

Alcohol violation rate = (confirmed positives + refusals) ÷ (screens + refusals)

The positive rate[10] does not include refusals. For drugs, it is the number of verified positives per the total number of specimens collected. For alcohol, it is the total number of confirmed positives per the total number of screens collected.

5.1 Official Random Violation Rates from 1996 through 2002

As mentioned in Section 2.3, the combined percentage of positives plus refusals (i.e., the violation rate) is the best indication of the overall level of drug use and alcohol misuse, and is used by FTA in determining minimum random testing rates for the following year.

As shown in the following graph, the official drug violation rate rose in 2002, for the first time since employers in all size categories were required to report. The official weighted rate for 2002 rose above 1.0 percent, following its drop to 0.98 percent in 2001. Because the rate did not remain above 1.0 for a second consecutive year, the FTA Administrator did not have the option to reduce the

---

[10] For clarity in presenting the test results, the terms "violation rate" and "positive rate" are used differently in this report than in Part 655. See the text box in Section 2.3 for a full explanation.

drug test quota from 50 percent to 25 percent for 2003. Although the official drug violation rate rose by more than 7 percent in 2002, equaling the rate in 2000 of 1.05, it was still nearly 35 percent lower than the rate in 1996.

As also shown in the graph at right, the official random alcohol violation rate rose by more than 20 percent in 2002 (to 0.22 percent), equaling the highest rate (set in 1998). Despite its relatively high level, the 2002 alcohol violation rate remained well below the threshold of 0.50 percent for raising the testing rate from 10 to 25 percent.

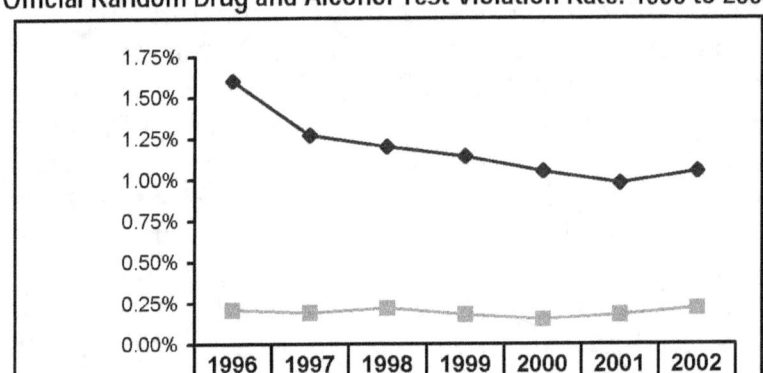

Official Random Drug and Alcohol Test Violation Rate: 1996 to 2002

	1996	1997	1998	1999	2000	2001	2002
Drugs	1.60%	1.27%	1.20%	1.14%	1.05%	0.98%	1.05%
Alcohol	0.21%	0.19%	0.22%	0.18%	0.15%	0.18%	0.22%

5.2 Actual Rates for Results Reported in 2001 and 2002

As shown in the graph below at left, both the transit and the contractor drug violation rates rose in 2002, reflecting the rise in the overall drug violation rate. The percentage of increase in the rate for transit employees was more than twice the percentage of increase for contractors. The alcohol violation rate for transit employees decreased while the rate for contractors increased.

As shown in the graph below at right, the combined positive drug test rate for random, post-accident, reasonable suspicion, and pre-employment tests remained the same, and the combined alcohol rate decreased.

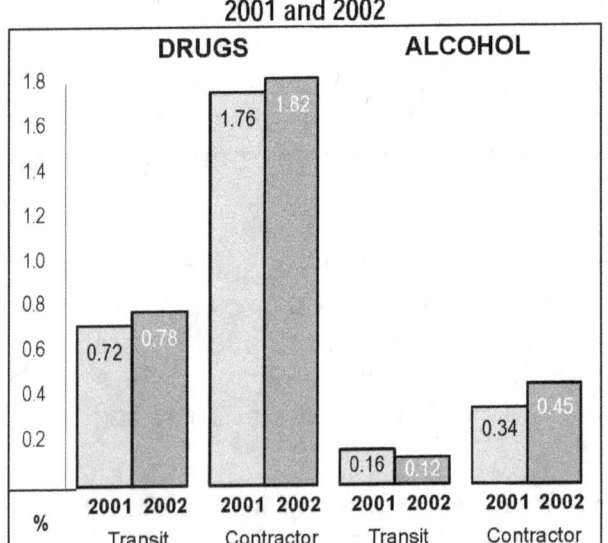

Actual Random Violation Rates by Employer Type: 2001 and 2002

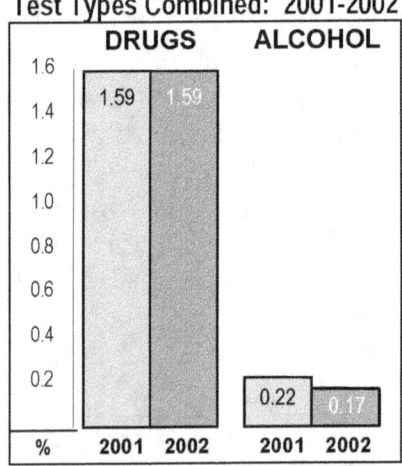

Actual Positive Rates for Four Test Types Combined: 2001-2002

Appendix A. Glossary

Accident: An occurrence associated with the operation of a vehicle, if as a result:

(1) A person dies;

(2) A person suffers a bodily injury and immediately receives medical treatment away from the scene of the accident;

(3) With respect to an occurrence in which the mass transit vehicle involved is a bus, electric bus, van, or automobile, one or more vehicles incurs disabling damage as the result of the occurrence and is transported away from the scene by a tow truck or other vehicle; or

(4) With respect to an occurrence in which the mass transit vehicle involved is a rail car, trolley car, trolley bus, or vessel, the mass transit vehicle is removed from revenue service.

Alcohol: The intoxicating agent in beverage alcohol, ethyl alcohol, or other low molecular weight alcohols including methyl or isopropyl alcohol.

Alcohol concentration: The alcohol in a volume of breath expressed in terms of grams of alcohol per 210 liters of breath as indicated by a breath test.

Alcohol confirmation test: A subsequent test using an EBT, following a screening test with a result of 0.02 or greater, that provides quantitative data about the alcohol concentration.

Alcohol positive: See "confirmed positive."

Screening test: An analytic procedure to determine whether an employee may have a prohibited concentration of alcohol in a breath or saliva specimen.

Alcohol use: The consumption of any beverage, mixture or preparation, including any medication containing alcohol.

Anti-drug program: A program to detect and deter the use of prohibited drugs as required by FTA regulations.

Armed security personnel: Function including any person who provides security to protect persons or property, and any person who carries a firearm.

Canceled or invalid test: In drug testing, a drug test that has been declared invalid by a Medical Review Officer (MRO). In alcohol testing, this would be a test that is deemed to be invalid. It is neither a positive nor a negative test.

CDL/non-revenue vehicle: Job category including any transit employee who holds a Commercial Driver's License (CDL), performs a function requiring a CDL, and is not included in any other job category.

Confirmed positive: A specimen with a confirmed breath alcohol level of at least 0.04

Consortium: An entity, including a group or association of employers, operators, recipients, subrecipients, or contractors, which provides drug testing services and acts on behalf of the employer.

Contractor: A person or organization that provides a service for a recipient, subrecipient, employer, or operator consistent with a specific understanding or arrangement. The understanding can be a written contract or an informal arrangement that reflects an ongoing relationship between the parties.

Covered employee: A person, including an applicant, transferee, and certain volunteers who perform a safety-sensitive function for a recipient, subrecipient, employer, or operator.

DOT: United States Department of Transportation.

DOT agency: An agency (or "operating administration") of the U.S. Department of Transportation administering regulations requiring drug testing.

Drug confirmation (or confirmatory) test: A second analytical procedure performed on a urine specimen to identify and quantify the presence of a specific drug or drug metabolite.

Drug metabolite: The specific substance produced when the human body metabolizes a given prohibited drug as it passes through the body and is excreted in urine.

Drug positive: See "verified positive."

Drug screening test (or initial test): An immunoassay screen of a urine specimen (collected in accordance with 49 CFR Part 40 and analyzed in a DHHS-approved laboratory), to eliminate "negative" urine specimens from further analysis. Positive specimens are analyzed again (via a confirmation test) to verify and quantify the presence of a specific drug or drug metabolite.

Education: Efforts that include the display and distribution of informational materials, a community service hotline telephone number for employee assistance, and the transit entity policy regarding drug use and alcohol misuse in the workplace.

Employee: A person designated in a DOT agency regulation as subject to drug testing and/or alcohol testing. "Employee" includes an applicant for employment.

Employer: A recipient or other entity that provides mass transportation services or performs a safety-sensitive function for such recipient or other entity. This term includes subrecipients, operators, and contractors.

Follow-up test: Required of employees who have returned to duty in a safety-sensitive position following a positive drug test result or an alcohol test result of ≥ 0.04. A minimum of six tests must be performed during the first 12 months after the employee returns to duty.

FTA: The Federal Transit Administration, an agency of the U.S. Department of Transportation.

Large operator: A recipient or subrecipient primarily operating in an area with a population of 200,000 or more.

Medical review officer (MRO): A licensed physician (Doctor of Medicine or Doctor of Osteopathy) responsible for receiving laboratory results generated by an employer's drug testing program, who has knowledge of substance abuse disorders and has appropriate medical training to interpret and evaluate a person's confirmed positive test result together with appropriate medical history and any other relevant biomedical information.

Part 40: US DOT's testing regulation titled *Procedures for Transportation Workplace Drug and Alcohol Testing Programs*, which was enacted in 1994 and revised in 2000.

Part 655: FTA's testing regulation titled *Prevention of Alcohol Misuse and Prohibited Drug Use in Transit Operations*. In was enacted in 2001 to expand the minimum requirements of the revised Part 40 and to combine the previous FTA testing regulations enacted in 1994: Part 653, *Prevention of Prohibited Drug Use in Transit Operations*, and Part 654, *Prevention of Alcohol Misuse in Transit Operations*.

Positive test rate: Used in this report, for clarity in presenting the test results, to refer to the number of confirmed alcohol positives per total number of screens collected or the number of verified drug positives per total number of specimens collected. This definition differs from the regulatory definition (in Part 655), where "positive rate" refers to the number of drug test positives and refusals combined per person selected to take a random test.

Post-accident testing: Required testing for prohibited drugs and alcohol, following certain mass transit accidents. These accidents include those in which a death occurs, medical treatment away from the scene is required, or one or more of the vehicles involved incurs disabling damage.

Pre-employment testing: Testing that is designed to identify applicants who have consumed a prohibited drug in the recent past. Employers are prohibited from hiring an applicant for a safety-sensitive function unless they have a verified negative drug test.

Random testing: Identifies employees who are using drugs or misusing alcohol by using an unpredictable and unannounced testing pattern. Safety-sensitive employees are selected based on a scientifically valid random-number selection method. It is considered by FTA to be the most effective deterrent to drug use and alcohol misuse.

Random testing rate: The rate at which each employer must conduct random tests each year. The number of random drug tests must equal a percentage (specified by FTA each year) of the number of the employer's safety-sensitive employees. In 2001, the drug testing rate was 50 percent, and the alcohol testing rate was 10 percent. These rates remained the same in 2002. They can be amended (per Part 655.45) by the FTA Administrator based on the combined percentage of positive tests plus test refusals.

Reasonable suspicion testing: Required when an employer has reasonable suspicion that an employee has used a prohibited drug or has misused alcohol as defined in the regulations. Reasonable suspicion testing must be based on specific, contemporaneous, articulable observations made by a trained supervisor concerning the appearance, behavior, speech, or body odor of a safety-sensitive employee.

Recipient: An entity receiving financial assistance under Section 5307, 5309, or 5311 of the Federal Transit Act or under Section 103(e)(4) of Title 23 of the U.S. Code. A *direct recipient* receives funding directly from FTA, i.e., most large transit agencies, state governments, and metropolitan planning organizations (MPOs). An in*direct recipient* receives funding from a state government or from an MPO.

Refusal to submit to an alcohol test: A covered employee fails to provide adequate breath for testing without a valid medical explanation.

Refusal to submit to a drug test: A covered employee fails to provide a urine sample as required by 49 CFR Part 40, without a valid medical explanation, after the employee has received notice of the requirement to be tested or engages in conduct that clearly obstructs the testing process.

Return to duty testing: Required before an employee is allowed to return to duty to perform a safety-sensitive function following a verified positive drug test, an alcohol result of 0.04 or greater, a refusal to submit to a test, or any other violation of the regulation.

Revenue vehicle control/dispatching: Job function including any person who controls the dispatch or movement of revenue service vehicles.

Revenue vehicle operations: Function including any person who operates or works as a crewman on revenue service vehicles at any time.

Rural operator: A subrecipient of 5311 funding primarily operating in an area with a population of less than 50,000.

Safety-sensitive function: Any of the following duties:

- Operating a revenue service vehicle, including when not in revenue service;
- Operating a non-revenue service vehicle, when required to be operated by a holder of a Commercial Driver's License (CDL);
- Controlling dispatch or movement of a revenue service vehicle;
- Maintaining a revenue service vehicle or equipment used in revenue service, unless the recipient receives section 5311 funding and contracts out such services; and/or
- Providing security and carrying a firearm.

Small operator: A recipient or subrecipient primarily operating in an area with a population of 50,000 or greater and less than 200,000.

Substance abuse professional (SAP): A licensed physician (Doctor of Medicine or Doctor of Osteopathy), or a licensed or certified psychologist, social worker, employee assistance professional, or addiction counselor (certified by the National Association of Alcoholism and Drug Abuse Counselors Certification Commission), with knowledge of and clinical experience in the diagnosis and treatment of drug and alcohol-related disorders.

Transit agency: The public entity that receives the Federal grant (direct grant recipient), whether or not that recipient provides mass transit services directly.

Vehicle and equipment maintenance: Function including any person repairing or maintaining revenue service vehicles or other equipment used in revenue service.

Verified positive: A drug test result reviewed by an MRO and determined to have evidence of prohibited drug use.

Violation rate: Used in this report, for clarity in presenting the test results, to refer to the number of test positives and refusals combined per person selected to take a random test:

Drug violation rate = (verified positives + refusals) ÷ (specimens collected + refusals)

Alcohol violation rate = (confirmed positives + refusals) ÷ (screens collected + refusals)

This definition differs from the regulatory definition (in Part 655), where "violation rate" refers only to alcohol testing. The concept of a drug violation rate is referred to as the "positive rate" in Part 655.

Appendix B. FTA Regions

The Federal Transit Administration (FTA) has ten regions, which are identified below. The data provided by these regions have facilitated the comparison of drug and alcohol test results and the identification of regional trends.

U.S. States and Territories Reporting to the 10 FTA Regions

Region 1	Region 2	Region 3	Region 4	Region 5
Connecticut	New Jersey	Delaware	Alabama	Illinois
Maine	New York	District of	Florida	Indiana
Massachusetts	Virgin Islands	Columbia	Georgia	Michigan
New Hampshire		Maryland	Kentucky	Minnesota
Rhode Island		Pennsylvania	Mississippi	Ohio
Vermont		Virginia	North Carolina	Wisconsin
		West Virginia	Puerto Rico	
			South Carolina	
			Tennessee	

Region 6	Region 7	Region 8	Region 9	Region 10
Arkansas	Iowa	Colorado	American Samoa	Alaska
Louisiana	Kansas	Montana	Arizona	Idaho
New Mexico	Missouri	North Dakota	California	Oregon
Oklahoma	Nebraska	South Dakota	Guam	Washington
Texas		Utah	Hawaii	
		Wyoming	Nevada	
			Northern	
			Mariana Islands	

Appendix C.
Accident and Fatality Data Associated with Positive Post-Accident Tests by FTA Region

As mentioned in Section 3.2, the number of accidents in which a transit agency employee or contractor tested positive in an FTA post-accident test cannot be expressed as a rate, and the data reported cannot be normalized by FTA region. The number of accidents, fatal accidents, and total fatalities that were reported are presented by region in the table at right. The numbers for non-fatal accidents are subdivided by employer type and by employer size, respectively, in the two tables below. Because no fatal accidents were reported in 2001, the columns with fatality data are not included in those tables.

Accidents and Fatalities Resulting in Post-Accident Positives by FTA Region

Region	Drugs			Alcohol		
	Non-Fatal Accidents	Fatal Accidents	Total Fatalities	Non-Fatal Accidents	Fatal Accidents	Total Fatalities
1	4	0	0	0	0	0
2	19	0	0	0	0	0
3	24	0	0	0	0	0
4	8	0	0	0	0	0
5	30	0	0	4	0	0
6	6	0	0	0	0	0
7	4	0	0	0	0	0
8	7	0	0	0	0	0
9	19	1	1	0	0	0
10	5	0	0	0	0	0

It should be noted that one person may test positive for both drugs and alcohol and that most employers test the employee for both drugs and alcohol. Thus, the numbers for drugs and alcohol cannot be added to obtain the total number of persons who tested positive. Data were not reported on the total number of persons testing positive in a post-accident test or for persons testing positive for both drugs and alcohol.

Non-Fatal Accidents Resulting in Post-Accident Positives by FTA Region and Employer Type

Region	Drugs		Alcohol	
	Transit	Contractor	Transit	Contractor
1	3	1	0	0
2	9	10	0	0
3	9	15	0	0
4	7	1	0	0
5	23	7	4	0
6	4	2	0	0
7	4	0	0	0
8	0	7	0	0
9	9	10	0	0
10	4	1	0	0

Non-Fatal Accidents Resulting in Post-Accident Positives by FTA Region and Employer Size

Region	Drugs			Alcohol		
	Large	Small	Rural	Large	Small	Rural
1	4	0	0	0	0	0
2	19	0	0	0	0	0
3	24	0	0	0	0	0
4	4	3	1	0	0	0
5	30	0	0	4	0	0
6	6	0	0	0	0	0
7	4	0	0	0	0	0
8	7	0	0	0	0	0
9	19	0	0	0	0	0
10	3	0	2	0	0	0